950

YO-CDA-529

FROM WHY TO YES

ain Uncovers the
leaningful Life to a
hilosopher

oseph H. Casey

VERSITY
SS OF
ERICA

LANHAM • NEW YORK • LONDON

Copyright © 1982 by

University Press of America,™ Inc.

4720 Boston Way
Lanham, MD 20706

3 Henrietta Street
London WC2E 8LU England

Library of Congress Cataloging in Publication Data

Casey, Joseph H.
    From why to yes.

    1. Casey, Joseph H. 2. Catholic Church–Clergy–
Biography. 3. Clergy–United States–Biography. 4.
Pulmonary embolism–Patients–United States–
Biography. 5. Suffering. I. Title.
BX4705.C335727A34   282'.092'4 [B]   81–43471
ISBN 0–8191–2205–X (pbk.)   AACR2

Dedicated

with affectionate gratitude

to

all those whose caring

protected me.

Contents

v

CHAPTER ONE

Pain, Tears and PAIN

I sense a lack of meaning in the lives of many whom I meet and of all ages. "I wish I were in the box" one elderly lady blurted out after a year in a rest home. "I am white, middle-class, formally educated through the M.A. degree, employed in a large corporation. I earn something in the order of $20,000 a year, have my own home, two cars, have been twice married, twice in therapy, etc. etc., etc. And I hate it. All of it. There is no meaning in any of this. And now as I approach middle life...I find nothing is stable, nothing is true." Thus a business man a few years ago. Old, middle aged and young as well. The disenchantment of the young spawned the counter-culture a few years ago. Economic pressures may have muted the challenge to established values. But in the hearts of many still lurks the question--Is there really any meaning to all this?

My heart resonates with such bewilderment and suffering. For a few years ago life lost its meaning for me. After some months, meaning returned and I wanted once again to live and to work. But I am humbly aware, and frightened, that I had little control over any part of the process. I do not know what might cause me to lose heart again.

I want to share my experience. The pain, the loss of meaning may make us brothers. The return of meaning may reassure. The anguish gave birth to new insights into meaning. While ideas will not restore meaning, they may stir those in darkness to seek their own understanding. The effort to do so can help in the process of recovering meaning. These insights may provide hints to the young as they strive to build meaningful lives and serve others as means to assess symptoms of lack of meaning in their lives. Let me tell you what happened.

August 27, 1969 changed my life. I had experienced little sickness or real pain during my life. In the next three months I was to discover a gamut running from sharp, surface pain to deep, throbbing discomfort to shocking black pain of horror. This last took meaning out of my life.

1

It began that Monday morning when the house phone startled me out of sleep. "Are you planning to say Mass for us?" A week previously I had agreed to say Mass at a nearby girls' college but had forgotten. Now a nun was phoning me from the front door. I dressed hastily and dashed downstairs. A modishly dressed woman, the nun, was sitting at the wheel of an old car. With my apology and a futile effort to fasten the seat belt we were off. As we rounded the first sharp curve, Sister reached over to help me find the ashtray but stiffened and cried "It won't turn" as the car raced straight ahead onto the lawn. I looked at her in dismay and leaned over to force the wheel around. I never thought to yell "brake" or to turn off the ignition. We hit the tree. (I am so conscious of that tree each time I pass it now.)

I felt nothing. I had blacked out. Terrible bruises witnessed to the tossing and beating I must have taken. Moments later I heard Sister crying, "My knee... my knee. Oh, Father, I'm sorry." I leaned over in an instinctive response to help. But I could not get over to her. With the momentum of the effort I turned back to the door, pushed myself out and screamed for help.

I entered the school of pain. Pain would teach me the realities of life--in two hard lessons. In the first, pain would instruct strictly, severely, but gentlemanly, searing but not gashing. Pain would attack as a destroyer in the second lesson two months later.

Lying on the ground my screams brought help. Grace Allen rushed out of the house as we crashed in her driveway. Cars stopped. Jesuits from the college heard and responded. No one would yield to my plea to shift my body to relieve the pain in my leg and hip. But Grace had her son bring me a pillow for my head. As they lifted me into the police cruiser I heard shouted directives to wait for a firetruck to pry Sister out of the car. Racing to the hospital I felt I had to hold on for dear life as I swayed back and forth.

The doctor at the emergency entrance to the Waltham Hospital wasted no time. Walking beside the stretcher he shot questions at me. Where do you hurt? Who is your doctor? Do you want any particular doctor at the hospital? Somebody, I still do not know who, stated firmly that Dr. Guiney had been asked to handle both Sister and myself. Surprised but assuming some one had good reasons for the choice I kept silent. After further questions specific X-rays were ordered.

From the examining room they wheeled me into the corridor of the X-ray department. The leg and hip hurt intensely. Again I sought something like a pillow to prop up my leg. Girls in white sped by but ignored my pleas, powerless as they rightly were to put sympathy before medical procedure. Finally the doctor who had admitted me came along and provided a pillow. The X-ray technician greeted me with warm concern, for she had been a penitent of mine at St. Julia's Church in Weston. After wheeling me into the dark room she had me lifted onto the cold table; her presence gave me confidence even while she hurt me more by pushing me into the contorted positions needed for the X-rays the doctor had ordered. Only after these were checked did the needle sink into my hip and blot out the pain.

The drug took effect almost instantly. I knew nothing of the elevator trip to the third floor. A blurred image remains of my entering the room which was to be my home and classroom for three months. It was a large, private room at the end of a side corridor outfitted with the latest equipment.

A mild concussion prevented the operation on the hip until Wednesday. During these two days as well as a few days after the operation I was heavily medicated. There was considerable pain. I recall asking often for the needle and when the shoulder hurt from the shots, I asked for oral administration. I soon went back to the needle.

I do not recall anything about the operation on the hip, not even being prepared for it. The ascetabulum was the trouble spot. The hip was pinned. This meant no cast was needed, but the leg was in traction for six weeks. Symbolically I too was suspended in air.

Pain continued. I was too weak and sore to feed myself. My brother Ed and his wife Miriam came daily and fed me supper. Mary and Tom, my sister and her husband, also came daily. I cried easily and this distressed me until a doctor friend whom I phoned for explanation reassured me that this was a common physiological reaction to the shock of an operation. During the six weeks I frequently experienced humiliating dependence. So often words of apology started to my lips. I never spoke them. I sensed to do so would be to apologize for being human.

Thus far my first lesson in pain. Pain was a severe instructor but it did not penetrate or cut to the

heart. I learned life but was able to come to grips
with it. My recollections of these days summon up the
picture of a faith quite operative. Somehow I sensed
that Christ was suffering in and through me. There was
no rebellion or resentment. I tried to read parts of
the gospels. I could not really pray, it seemed, but
there were repeated flashes of faith. I recall a strong
sense that sickness is evil and that Christ's role as
well as the role of Christians was not primarily to bear
it but to overcome it. On other occasions swift reflections came that prayer grows out of living and that I
should be primarily concerned to live as a Christian
faced with suffering--and let prayer grow out of this.
I lacked, of course, the energy to read or think or
pray. It was a question of survival with flashes of
prayerful insight. However these observations are not
pious reflections. They do, I believe, capture the attitude with which I faced life in these circumstances.

The days became more interesting as the pain
ceased, discomfort lessened and my strength crept back.
The dark room ceased to spread gloom, yielding to the
brightening of flowers, of cards stretched across the
wall, but especially to the warm smiles of loving
friends. The day came when I was able to get out of
bed and sit up. I still remember my favorite nurse,
Sue Tepper, my "wigged one," getting me on my feet for
the first time. I had gone through the procedure many
times in imagination, planning each movement with apprehension. The smoothness of her technique and her
respect for my fears impressed me. Finally into a
wheelchair, down on the elevator to the physio-therapy
department. Just to enter that room brightened the
day. I really liked the girls there. (Later I offici-
ated at three of their weddings). I used to joke with
my lovely blond therapist, Vivian McDonald, that she
should tell her fiancée that I ached for her every
night. Vivian introduced me to crutches, exercised my
legs with weights and my arms as well. Pains and aches
in arm muscles, shoulders, back and chest were regular.

The end was in sight. The doctor told me I could
leave the hospital within a week of my birthday, October 13. It would be almost two months. Although pro-
spects seemed bright two things signalled warnings.
Besides the pains and aches mentioned earlier there was
the growing resentment I experienced. I felt the nurs-
es were taking advantage of me, neglecting my needs as
I began to recover. So keenly did I feel this that
when they brought in a cake at lunch and sang "Happy
Birthday" I coldly acknowledged it, but refused to

touch the cake. I was not going to allow this hospital
any share in my birthday. In retrospect I presume cir-
culatory problems were basic to my reactions. For the
pains and aches were far more than I later experienced
when I took up crutches again and such resentment was
not normal for me nor did it recur.

Ironically the end of lesson one fused with the
start of lesson two in a bright party on my fifty-second
birthday. Friends streamed in. Mary and Tom brought
me a lobster dinner. Someone else brought a cake. Since
the location of my room lessened the likelihood of dis-
turbing other patients, the room was full till late.

Trouble began that night. It started with muscle
aches and pains, moved to what I interpreted as a muscle
wrench but what was actually pulmonary embolism. To relieve the aches I asked for a heatpack. I had it first
on my chest, then on my back. When I tried to remove
it I thought I pulled a muscle. The pain was severe.
The superb night nurse, worried, summoned the superin-
tendent since no orders were on the books for pain medication. I was reluctant to have them phone the doctor,
especially since he was substituting for my regular doctor who had gone off for a vacation. Finally they did
phone at 6 a.m. He prescribed demerol which brought relief. In fact after the morning wash I sat up through
lunch. I decided to get back into bed by myself and in
the process again wrenched (so I thought) a muscle caus-
ing the same considerable pain. Physiotherapy was out
of the question. Waves of pain swept in and out. In
the evening one of my friends in concern reported to
nurse Sue Tepper that I was in pain. She literally ran
to me. This I shall never forget. Unable to contact
my substitute doctor, Sue searched out a doctor on another floor and cajoled him into looking at me. He immediately put me on an anticoagulant and prescribed heavy
drugs. And so I entered a black tunnel.

I can recall the fact that I suffered intensely. I
cannot recall the emotion or the pain of that time. I
have to make an effort to recall this, for it slips away
into the past. What I see is blackness, a black tunnel
or even a black attacker. I do not reexperience the
pain, but remember only that it was the worst, the deepest I have ever had. The sharp, prolonged, penetrating
pain in the chest seemed to force all of me into one
point. I recall in the darkness uttering the challenge,
how could there be a God who would permit such pain. I
argued that as creator of the world He could have prevented such pain being possible. A dark night of black

5

physical pain and emotional shock. Another part of me
countered that charge with the image of the Son of God
dying on the cross. It was a counter, emotional shock
to that of the black doubt, for the mind could find no
clear, facile explanation of the initial challenge. Yet
even to this counter emotional shock I cried out I am
suffering more than Christ.

Pain became PAIN, attacking and destroying. How
long this blackness lasted I cannot be sure. About a
week, I believe, for the doctor found the symptoms contradictory. Finally the decision was reached to operate
on the venacava, plicating it. I drifted in and out of
this black period of pain and medication, alone, not
caring, without the energy to care what happened. I did
not face the proximity of death. It was limbo time, a
state not of desiring to survive, but of mere survival.

During the stressful days after the operation even
in my weakened state I built a new attitude toward pain.
Pain seemed now so horrible and the thing to be avoided.
The doctor ordered a catheter. The orderly tried to insert it, my cries prevented him. So the doctor came
with Sue Tepper and forced it in over my cries. I had
become so sensitive to pain. Indeed I felt embarrassed
my little friend should see me so babyish. Airplanes,
it flashed to me, should hold no fear for me, since
death in any accident would be too swift for much pain.
The picture of my father dying a year before from emphysema came to mind. During his last days I had felt he
was so lonely, life held little happiness for him. Why
not die, and if emphysema kept him from living through
more such, more power to emphysema. Very dispassionate-
ly it seemed clear to me that I did not want to live
long. Pain was the thing to be avoided. I wonder if I
shall always be fearing that any future pain will re-
semble the depth of the black, attacking pain of the embolism.

PAIN had taught its lesson. The effects were still
to be realized. I cried easily, I recall. My outlook
was not bitter, but tinged with cynicism. I understood
why people wanted to die. Enthusiasms struck me as
shallow, shared only by people not living the real. I
seldom prayed. I did not read scripture. My reception
of Holy Communion was perfunctory.

As I began to mend and my strength grew I think I
found the presence and love of family and dear friends,
the numerous cards, letters, flowers and gifts from
other friends and acquaintances a subtle support. The

pain had shocked me emotionally, deeply in my faith. The emotional appeal to the crucifixion countering this shock found support in the love I experienced. Neither the thought of the crucifixion nor the love banished the effect of the pain. But they countered and arrested it.

Increased strength did not radically alter the mood. As I moved back into the physio-therapy and practice on the crutches, I did what had to be done. Muscular aches and pains plagued me, but not nearly so much as before. There was no eagerness as I awaited the day of discharge. I looked ahead to difficulties coping with such situations as the long walk to the dining room and the heavy elevator doors. There was no eagerness, neither was there reluctance. Just a not-caring attitude, I guess. It was a dull period, for my energies were low, physically, emotionally, spiritually. There was pleasure when special friends came, but little joy in my life.

Thanksgiving week, three months after my accident, brought departure day. I was not excited. A doctor friend drove me home. Apprehension tightened me at every corner. To reassure me he reminded me he had driven his wife to the hospital four times with child and mother and infant home each time safely. I smiled and did relax a little. A room on the first floor had been well prepared for me and it was nice to move in.

Fellow Jesuits welcomed me in an uneffusive, genuine, fraternal way. I was at home. Special needs were provided for. The long walk on crutches to the dining room proved to be taxing. Too weak to open the elevator doors I had to wait patiently until someone came along. I started to weave back into my normal patterns. Fresh air tasted and felt so good. Sitting outside I discovered the sky is blue. It was not the experience of recalling or rediscovering. It felt like discovering. I had to rebuild many elements in the framework of my life. But life consisted in eating, sleeping, awkward crutching about, not much reading, visiting with friends.

None of this was distasteful. Indeed being with friends was very pleasant. But nothing was important. I heard no call to anything. I had moved into a state of unmeaningful existence. It was not a painful or nauseous state. But nothing really gripped me, nothing struck me as important. Nothing was I keenly alert, keenly desirous to achieve.

In fact it was with a sort of distanced amazement

that I watched anyone earnest or eager about anything.
I recognized how important to President Nixon were his
proposals as I watched him speak to the nation on T.V.
The intense efforts of performers to put across their
numbers came through to me. The commitment of the 'Vin-
veremos', American volunteers, to harvest Cuban sugar
cane, impressed me. To me nothing was important. I
heard no call to anything.

PAIN caused this. Somehow it shook the center of
my soul and produced this unmeaningful mood. Later I
shall try to understand what happened and why, but first
let me finish describing my experience.

I can, of course, speak only about the conscious
level. I do not know what transpired on the unconscious
level or on the physiological. Without doubt the physiological, hormonal change due to the operation and pain
left me with less energy, less inclination or ability to
get excited. And as my body rebuilt its energy no doubt
the opposite had a definite influence. Still there definitely was a psychological element. For things
seemed different when I changed spiritually.

Blending together and, I suspect, mutually nurturing each other were three decisive elements. Jesus became real to me again. The whole of life, history and
the universe began once more to make sense. And I
seemed called to a role in the world plan.

Something special stirred in me as I celebrated
Mass in my room the day I returned from the hospital.
It was the first Mass in three months and close friends
attended. Each day I sat at a small table to do the
same, not, of course, with the special stirring. Soon
I was drawn to spend a few minutes daily just attending
to God's presence within me--with but modest results.
I cannot explain to you how I could do this if God had
become unimportant to me. I lived on habit, custom,
not desire. And pain had not swept me into disbelief.

The Mass and personal prayer recreated to some extent the sense of the reality of God, but they were far
from effecting any radical change in my outlook of unmeaningful existence. Around Christmas time awareness
of my mood sharpened when the Superior asked me to direct a weekend retreat for a college boy. Spontaneously I accepted but second thoughts surged up as I recognized how uncommitted I was. Was it fair to the boy to
speak about a Christ who was so unimportant to me? Perhaps Divine Providence had it that no one else was

available. Preparing for the retreat laid the ground-
work for my recovery.

I got hold of my retreat notes which I had reworked
the preceding January with a new focus upon Scripture,
especially St. Paul. Two reactions were significant as
I reread my talks. St. Paul's utter conviction that
Jesus Christ had directly called him impressed me again.
Secondly, Paul's vision of God's plan to restore all
things in Christ once more caught my attention.

Still nothing really happened within me to change
my outlook. Weeks were to pass before I began to make
headway. One more preliminary event somehow seems to
have mattered. I visited my Old Aunt Min in a conva-
lescent home in Lynn. She was dear to me, a beautiful,
gentle, self-effacing person with a gift of simple
laughter. But she was too weak to speak. Still I sensed she realized my sister, Mary, and I were there.
Within a week Min had died.

Some weeks later my mind started to probe the meaning of life. Perhaps because my trouble had started
with pain, perhaps because I was living with old and
sick men, perhaps because of Aunt Min my efforts to find
meaning in life began by trying to make sense out of
suffering, growing old and dying.

Paul's words flashed to mind: "I live, now not I,
but Christ lives within me." With such a belief one
was not alone in facing these terrible experiences. God
would be experiencing them within me. Indeed in a certain sense God needed me to experience them as I did.
Such reflections at this point were only ideas. No
commitment was involved. I was but tentatively weighing
the fact that belief in Christ would give meaning to
suffering, aging and death. Death would lose its terror
for it would become the doorway to life with Our Lord
for eternity.

But as I focused upon Christ as the source of providing meaning, I felt the need of far more than the
making sense of suffering, growing old and dying. I
needed to understand what the meaning and/or purpose of
the universe and mankind is. I was concerned about the
development of the universe. Those were days of demonstrations, marches and general revolutionary ideas.
Young revolutionaries wanted radical changes in society.
So many priests, ministers, seminarians and religious
were engaging in direct social action. Many were also
committing themselves to restructuring the church and/or

their religious orders. The power of organized effort was bursting as an accepted insight upon groups in all areas of life and tactical maneuvering and manipulating became almost a game.

So much that was going on I admired. The determined movement of the Blacks to achieve their rights and their dignity. The dedication of their leaders as well as the whites who actively supported them. The ambitions of the New Left to reorder the priorities in our country and alleviate the sufferings of the poor. The focus of the hippies on the values of love, of enjoyment in present activities and freedom rather than drudgery and postponement of enjoyment for the sake of economic success to the point of shriveling up as a human being. The fusion of all these movements in the peaceful demonstrations for peace with the growing abhorrence of war and its evils.

But as I observed commitment in these various forms--aware as well of the harmful aspects--I recaptured the realization that Jesus Christ grounded all the good in these movements. The preceding summer, for example, as I drove around the poor section of Asheville, North Carolina, and realized how terribly hot it must be in some of those houses of the poor, I reflected that had I money and my sister were living in such conditions I would insure she got better quarters. Now if I truly believe that Jesus Christ is living in and with these poor, I should be at least equally motivated to improve those terrible conditions.

In St. Paul we read God's plan sweeping through the centuries started with man's destiny to subdue and govern the earth so that humanization of the universe was the goal. But this was transformed by the incarnation of God in Jesus Christ. Men now would push toward their goal with Jesus Christ. In fact men could not become fulfilled as men except through and in and with Jesus Christ. Instead of humanizing men must Christmanize the universe. Christ instituted--and his followers are to continue--a transcendent critique of all human enterprises. Whatever is human is to be pursued and all form of human institutions are to be challenged by the message of Christ. "Challenged"?--not only challenged but transformed by the life and power Jesus has brought into the world of men.

Christian theistic humanism, interpreted as I have with the aid of St. Paul, provides an overarching meaning to life which responds to every desire for human betterment which the most revolutionary propose. It grounds these desires in the deepest truths, warns against the abuses so often accompanying these movements, and carries with it the life and power to achieve what is envisioned.

These were not new ideas for me but a recovery of the outlook I previously operated with taking shape afresh as I probed for meaning. Two points are essential for understanding what was taking place in me. Stating these broad ideas might suggest that speculative reflection was the key, but it was lived encounter with Jesus Christ which mattered. Scripture explaining who and what Jesus Christ is whom one encounters together with the Church's interpreting of Christ's message for our day were needed and shaping. But they fused into the experience of the living reality of Jesus Christ.

I did not think my way out of my depression. Jesus Christ came to me, touched me. I am not suggesting any extraordinary or mystical experience. As I celebrated Mass and entered into quiet prayer gradually it became real for Jesus became real for me once again. Somehow I sensed His presence within me. Faith interpreted the subjective experience and I just knew it was Christ. For this reason the intellectual understanding of the meaning of life took on vibrant conviction from the living person of Christ.

The second essential point is that I sensed I was being called by Christ, needed by Him in a specific role. Mankind needed Christ, needed His life and power for its fulfillment. Christ's Church as the carrier of that life then was needed. And there was something I could contribute both as priest and as the person I am at this critical period of history.

I was not sure just why or in what role Christ wanted me. Perhaps He could use me as one of the mediators in this period of change. Never radical enough to initiate the correcting of situations harmful to men, neither was I zealously aware of and committed to preserving values achieved and incarnated in our institutions. Rather I am among the third group open to change yet appreciative of the old. Change will not be effected without people of the radical 'left'; change will be destructive without the people of the radical 'right'; change will not be viable without the people of the middle. Perhaps God would use me as one of these mediators. On the other hand maybe Our Lord had something

else for me to do. I did not know. I did experience a
sense that he wanted me for who I am. I am not profes-
sing a dramatic or radical reconversion which fired me
with enthusiasm and launched me on a rapid road to sanctity. But over a period of time meaning returned to my
life. I did become whole again and to the measure I was
able to be Jesuit priest, I felt liberated, joyful, effective. I felt confident I was on the path God wanted
me to follow and each day at Mass I offered myself to
God, hoping that some day I might mean it effectively.
In the meantime I was trying to allow the Blessed Trinity to live through me, to bring love, joy, help to
those I met. I tried to live and enjoy the present,
rather than strain or live only for the future. I tried
to bring my specific, even though limited contribution
to the communities I share: speculative reflection and
a blend of openness to change and concern to preserve
essentials.

This rebirth of meaning in my life was as gradual
and undramatic, but as profound as the rebirth of spring
in which it occurred. It was with desire that I now
laid plans for the coming academic year. That of 1969-
70 was to have been a sabbatical. In preparation for it
I had used the summer to outline a book I ambitioned
writing during the year. The accident turned the year
into a leave of absence and 1970-71 was to be my sabbatical. While life was unmeaningful I faced the prospect of a year away with no desire. Writing a book was
out of the question. With the rebirth of meaning desires returned. Friends helped me to arrange a fellow-
ship at Yale Divinity and find a room in the Ecumenical
Continuing Education Center at Yale.

I settled into my new home at the end of August.
It was a very large bedroom-study with bath on the dark
but quiet rear corner of the Center. Out came the outline for the book, but I found myself reflecting on
what had happened to me, very much aware that had meaning not returned I would not have been there. It seemed
right that I should describe and explain what happened
and insert it as a foreword. More than being 'right'
it felt as though it might help the many others facing
life without meaning.

My state of non-meaningful existence was not painful, but prolonged living without meaning might gradually lead to a sense of meaningless existence, which,
in its painfulness, would raise what Camus claimed to
be the only real question--suicide. Many of our young,
I fear, are facing such experience. We wonder why they

'cop out', why education, so important for their future, is so often rejected. The goals and values of the 'establishment' generation which do make education important in many cases no longer appeal, no longer call to them as important. Inanition is avoided because the energy of youth drives them on for immediate pleasures and satisfactions. They start running, distracting themselves from ultimate questions. Laughter for such can be witless distraction, a cover-up, an escape, perhaps even a ritual reminder that laughter itself may produce the interior contentment and enjoyment it normally symbolizes. Unfortunately pursuit of the immediate can lead the young to taste the bitter dregs of emptiness in alluring pleasures which tasted turn bitter. I have in mind young people like Janis Joplin. The New York Times carried this account of the rock singer's suicide: "Miss Joplin drank as she lived-- with an all-consuming intensity, as though she knew she did not have much time...Asked what she wanted out of life she replied, 'To be stoned, staying happy and having a good time. I'm doing just what I want with my life, enjoying it. When I get scared and worried I tell myself, "Janis, just have a good time". So I juice up real good and that's just what I have.'

Perhaps, I told myself, I can learn from my actual experience what makes a meaningful life and how meaning gets lost. If so I may be able to help our young as they struggle through these confused values to build meaningful and happy lives, I may be even more able to help people my own age who have lost meaning in their lives.

Foreword--Forebook

August 29, 1969 changed my life. August 1970 began one of the most satisfying years of my life. The
sabbatical proved to be healing--not because meaning
had returned to my life but because I came to grip with
the tensions of those years which were alienating and
painful to bear. Instead of picking up the work outlined the preceding summer I decided to devote the year
to settling mind and heart on the issues tearing me
apart in each of the communities to which I belonged.

Changes in the church, changes in the Society of
Jesus, changes in the university, radical changes in
civil society provoked anger, confusion, fear in the
hearts of most. Probing, letting surface what bother-
ed me, I crystalized for myself the areas of conflict
and distress, discovering they were the same in each of
my communities. A general, roughly drawn plan for the
year was soon realized. I would let emerge my spontaneous feelings on each of these trouble spots and then
assess my reactions in the light of reflected reexami-
nation of my fundamental beliefs. To shed light on my
reactions I sought insight into how I had come to be
the person I am, to hold the values I do. I focused
on the communities which shaped me starting with my family, the McClory-Casey community. This turn to the au-
tobiographical suggested how right it would be to describe in a foreword what happened the year before. So
serious an experience was bound to influence how I would
approach problems. As I labored to catch in words the
loss and rebirth of meaning, description failed to satisfy me. Just why did pain affect me that way? I had
to think my way through the experience. The foreword
grew and grew and became the Forebook.

Perhaps this may prove to be the most valuable effect of the experience. My reaction was not exception-
al. I believe it is referred to as reactive depression.
Having lived through the experience I might be able to
intuit the structure of a meaningful life from within
and to discover by reflection the elements that make it
up. Such efforts might providentially help others: the
many with the same experience of depression after pain,
those from whose lives the radical changes in church
and society have caused meaning to flee, the young who

15

today need guidelines for building their lives.

Each morning after breakfast I would sit at my desk to think and to write. "To think" meant to focus upon an issue, to taste, to reflect, to analyze, to wonder, to join all I knew. When I moved in the direction of the foreword it became clear I had to decide what meaningful meant. Does non-meaningful differ from meaningless? I hoped further that reflective analysis of my experience would uncover the essential elements constituting a meaningful life. If I could articulate by means of these elements just how pain destroyed the meaning in my life, I felt it would confirm my analysis.

Thus began an intellectual adventure. Really looking at my lived experience I let it reveal to me what had happened and what elements went into meaning in my life. The obvious difference between the way I now felt and the way I felt after the pain was the presence or absence of desires. Now I wanted to live, I desired to do things, things were important. Then nothing was important, I experienced no real desires. I did not think about wanting to live or not.

Anchored in simple description I sought light by linking my experience with two uses of the term "meaning" which I had often had to cope with. For years I had been grappling with a philosophical school of thought called Linguistic Analysis which viewed all of philosophy as a question of language. Such thinkers eliminated many traditional positions not as untrue by as 'meaningless'. God-talk, for instance, was not false. It just had no meaning. In the 1960's, on the other hand, secularizing and the 'Death of God' theologians proclaimed that all talk about God was 'meaningless' in the sense of irrelevant, unimportant. In my course on Philosophy and Religion I forced the challenge: Is God-talk semantically meaningless because it is irrelevant? Or is it meaningless, in the sense of irrelevant, because it is indeed semantically meaningless?

'Meaning' in one case refers to the intellect. Clues in detective stories, for instance are meaningful facts: they point beyond themselves. Or take this situation: John and Jim return to Jim's home after a day's work to find Jim's wife all dressed up with an excellent meal ready to be served. To John it is a factual situation. Jim may see far more: "I'm sorry," his wife is saying, "about our argument last night. Can we make up?" The facts point beyond themselves and only one who has the proper background or the correct perspective will see 'the beyond'. I am convinced that the analysts who rule out God-talk as semantically meaningless simply

16

lack the correct perspective to 'see the facts as' they are.

'Meaning' in the sense of relevance expresses a relation to the will. The young have recently insisted on meaning, on relevance in what they do. What they seem to intend primarily is not what 'makes sense', a relation to the intellect, but what grips a person, a relation to the will. I found students rejecting metaphysics as 'irrelevant' but exulting in the 'relevance' of 14th century French lyrics! The 'death of God' theologians were reporting that God and the transcendent had become unimportant to man, irrelevant. In this context 'meaning' refers to the appeal of the good, the valuable, the important, the desirable.

Applying this distinction to my experience it is 'meaning' in the sense of relevance that concerns me primarily. Yet a little probing uncovers a relation to the intellect as well. When I identified the difference between the way I now felt and the way I had felt after the pain as the presence or absence of desires I was focusing on the experience of activities appealing as good, as important. We might designate as meaningful in this sense whatever attracts, holds or drives one on. There is alertness, but also an element of the desirable and beneficial. Listening to a concert or engaged in loving conversation are examples. Deafening rock music would find me keenly alert but I would not find it meaningful, but something to flee.

To want a goal involves wanting the means. An activity then may not have intrinsic appeal but prove extrinsically meaningful. A particular college course may not in itself attract a person yet be recognized as a necessary means to a desired end and be very meaningful extrinsically. There is involved here a relation to the mind as well as to the will. The mind must recognize the relation. Taking this unattractive course must 'make sense'.

As I wondered recollecting the steps to the recovery of meaning in my life I found another reference to the intellect as I dwelt upon the days I searched to make sense out of suffering, aging, dying--indeed of the entire enterprise of the universe. The Pauline interpretation of God's plan to restore all things in Christ satisfied my search. It now struck me that a meaningful life required a presupposition of an intellectually satisfying nature that the whole of life made sense.

If all lives passed through a 'meaning' prism, at

one end would glow the intensely meaningful life, one which strongly attracts, holds, drives a person on. Near the middle would shine the contented life, which keeps one wanting to do what is needed to keep the pattern of life viable. The rest of the spectrum would go all the way through the lives of 'quiet desperation', those of drab overall meaning and occupied with lack-lustre activities, to those lives in which one hates or is appalled by all one does.

This prism image may allow me to identify what happened to me in terms of a shift in the spectrum. My life normally has been and is meaningful. Perhaps I should locate it between contentment and intensely meaningful. It lacked the intensity of the life of responsibility of a person like the President or like the doctor with a hospital full of patients dependent on him. There was not the keen alertness of the man in danger or conflict or high adventure. On the other hand beyond the state of contentment, characterized by satisfied overall meaning in life and a quiet habitual pattern of pleasing activities, I regularly had realistic goals with genuine, effective hope of achieving them. Pursuit of these goals involved recurrent periods of intense alertness and determination to achieve.

After the pain I would describe my life as non-meaningful and situate it below contentment but short of quiet desperation or the nauseous state of the meaningless. Nothing gripped me, nothing was important. I felt called to nothing. I was keenly alert about nothing. It was not that I had become quietly content. In contentment desire pulses beneath the habitual pattern of activities. Evidence of this is experienced in the distress or anger felt when one is prevented from doing them. I felt too dull to experience such distress or anger. Yet life had not become desperate, let alone absurd, nauseous, painful which I associate with the 'meaningless'. Hence I designate my state as non-meaningful.

Through such reflection the identification of my mood as non-meaningful stood forth. The temporal sequence of events was obvious. Life was meaningful. Severe pain. Life was non-meaningful. From the beginning I associated the emotional shock of doubt about God experienced at the time of the pain as pivotal. The emotional shock was countered by the emotional appeal of the crucifix supported subtly by the love friends gave. So it never reached denial of God's existence. In fact it was not even intellectual doubt summoning my mind to settle it. I simply no longer counted on God. I knew one concern: avoid pain. God ceased to be important to me.

This mood was a new experience. I had been unhappy before, sad before. This was different. I had even experienced unhappiness living with serious doubt about God's existence, but the very effort to resolve the doubt--one way or the other--kept life meaningful. Life cannot be happy without meaning. But life can be meaningful without being happy. When my life was shaken by those serious doubts I was unhappy and distressed. But I felt almost driven to face up to the challenge--is God real? Is Jesus Christ God? This engaged all of me. It was most meaningful.

Happiness, I sense, requires meaning, but is found in truth and wisdom. Meaning need not be truth--conviction suffices. But without truth happiness will suffer. Commitment to a life of crime or license may give meaning, but not happiness. Living in the truth but without wise provision for human needs will not bring happiness either.

Happiness is a very broad issue. My concern is about the core of happiness, meaning. I had identified my mood, I saw the sequence. In fact on one level the explanation was clear. God was central in my life. Speaking not piously or in terms of what ought to be but simply, honestly, the most satisfying experiences of my life as well as the most distressing have been related to God. While I have not lived a significantly good Jesuit life nor been a significantly good person, the drama of my personal life has focused not upon worldly success but upon my union with God. Shake the center of anyone's life and meaning dissolves. Little wonder life ceased to be meaningful when God ceased to count.

But it is precisely that little wonder which grew and moved me on. Just what is the relationship of God and meaning in my life? It was the pursuit of this problem that unveiled for me the constituent elements of meaning in any life, and these may prove enlightening to others. My position was privileged. When young we have no guarantee even wise choices will succeed in building a meaningful life. With no more wisdom than anyone else, I had been successful. When meaning was reborn to me it was indeed a rebirth, not a new discovery. By recollection and reflection I could detect the elements that blended into the single whole a meaningful life must be. Almost, as it were, from within I could intuit these elements, possessing an evidence that

19

no amount of mere speculation could equal.

What made possible this intuition from within was precisely recollection of the process of rebirth. Two essential elements emerged as blending into the restoration of the single whole. An overall answer to all the problems of life and the universe came to me which assured me that the whole of life was worth living. The "Good news" of Jesus Christ interpreted by St. Paul provided this answer for me. Later I was to discern that it was not the content but the fact that it provided some answer that made it a constitutive element of meaning. The second element was the harmonization I experienced in feeling Jesus Christ called me to a definite role in His work. Again further reflection let me see that it was the harmonization of my desires which mattered, not precisely the call of Christ.

So striking in the rebirth of meaning were these two elements that I could easily have ignored the contribution of other distinct elements. But the more I let my gaze range over the rest of my life the more the influence of these other elements stood out. While I imagine none of us ever lives on all the dimensions of his person, unless a sufficient number of key dimensions find expression, life will be dull. Women often experience monotony because in raising a family their intellectual curiosity and aesthetic inclinations receive no exercise. Meaning has been diminished in my life during periods when my activities were too restricted, but a more significant factor has been the extent of freedom and responsibility. The more I set goals and pursued them with responsibility, the more meaningful was my life. Grateful as I am for my Jesuit formation I believe I would have been more alive and developed if more choices had been mine.

Obviously meaning will be dependent upon a wise filling of one's life with activities which incarnate one's basic convictions, develop one's harmonized self, and at the same time allow as full expression of one's person as possible. This element of selecting activities ought not be taken for granted. A dull life often results from failure at this point.

Insight into the important role of freedom as well as the next two points I owe to the experience of meeting the counterculture of the 60's and early 70's. The NOW generation taught me that spontaneity is characteristic of life. Without it we are dead. What they warned me about was the unfreeing effects of habits and institutions. These latter strangely are also liberating. Without habits and institutions serving to provide nourishment, security, shelter and so forth, would we be 'free' to develop leisure, art, the intellectual life or even the critical appraisal of institutions? What happens, however, is that habits and institutions grow out of felt needs and desires, but tend to eliminate the feeling of need or desire, replacing it with a sense of "the next thing to be done" or even compulsion. Obviously spontaneity diminishes or dies. The raison d'etre of habits and institutions postulates a sensitivity to what is happening to oneself. Since their purpose is to liberate, so long as they liberate and provide room for spontaneity in important areas of living, they should be esteemed. When they shackle or dull, they should be changed.

The most serious threat to spontaneity that the counter-culture experienced was work. Our technocratic culture has so split up tasks, has so articulated the stages for the most efficient achievement of remote goals that most men find themselves employed in tasks which do not appeal, which do not engage enough of their talents, whose relation to those remote goals is not perceived, which goals themselves are often not worthwhile. How do you live spontaneously, "do your own thing" in such a culture? The conflict forced me to reflect on the "why" of work. Our sophisticated civilization so successfully provides for our basic needs that we often ignore their importance and priority. Actually everyone has to provide for the basic needs of food, shelter, security-- even in our society. The extrinsic appeal of so many jobs is that they bring the money which permits provision for the basic needs. What a difference if one can provide for basic needs by doing what one loves. The meaning in one's life will be definitely affected by the kind of work one does. The way it blends in with the source of one's personal harmonization of desires constitutes a major factor in the achievement of self-identity, meaning and happiness.

These are the elements I discovered in a meaningful life. A position which makes sense of the whole of life and the harmonization of desires are the two fundamental or central requisites. Provision for expression of a sufficient number of dimensions of one's person and responsible freedom definitely contribute as well. We often neglect to consider the element of a wise selection of activities expressive of the above. Living with habits and institutions, to the extent they liberate, yet sensitive to the shackling effects is another element. Finally the way one provides for basic needs and how this blends into the whole of one's life is very important.

Recollection and gazing on my experiences revealed this catalogue of elements constitutive of a meaningful life. Detection of the elements lured me to probe how these elements functioned to constitute meaning. I wanted understanding.

All that I am drove me to try to think through how these different elements blended and functioned. It took a college sophomore to let me see just what I was doing. In reaction to my experiences and explanation she wrote about meaning in her life. She had suffered much emotionally and mentally but had worked her way through to at least a very healthy start toward a happy life. For her the key had been the discovery that she had so admired and imitated her sister that she never let herself be herself. Once she started to grow from within, following her own desires and values she began to heal.

Many would, I believe, find her discovery more helpful than what I have to offer. Certainly basic to happiness is that one be oneself. A person has to know, esteem and love oneself to relate well and be happy. How one comes to know, esteem and love oneself may vary. Normally it requires a family of wise love. It seems fundamental that a person should grow from within. As years go on he becomes reflective upon the values, outlooks, positions he has been trained to and matures according as he accepts, rejects, or selects these with inner, personal conviction and desire. For the person who is confused or unhappy I can only urge personal assessment and determination to form one's own judgments of truth and value and to grow in free, responsible decisions.

What I attempted was not such practical analysis. I merely wanted to understand. If my reflections reveal the inner articulation of the elements of a meaningful life, they may help a person recognize what is lacking in his life. They will not suggest the process by which this lack may be corrected. If my reflections help anyone comprehend the construction of stages of developing meaning in one's life, they cannot <u>be</u> those stages. I am not suggesting a recipe for meaning and happiness. The individual has to incarnate these elements in a personal synthesis and adventure.

For a sick or unhappy person what matters is the cure or whatever makes one happy. There is no need to understand. On the other hand sometimes understanding frees one to develop one's own process. Underlying any technique or procedure to restore meaning or happiness must be the truth of all that is involved, whether known or not.

In any event the only thing I have to offer is my reflected understanding of how the constitutive elements in a meaningful life function. For myself I recall the genuine need I experienced to understand. Perhaps there are others who also crave understanding.

CHAPTER THREE

Overarching Meaning

In the rebirth of meaning which I had experienced the first hints of what was happening came with questions about the meaning of aging, sickness and dying. And these questions soon drove me to find an answer for life itself, history and the entire universe. Because of these experiences as well as the recognition that here I was touching one of the essential constituents of a meaningful life I had no hesitation where to begin.

It is important to keep in mind what my problem was at this point. I was not searching for the ultimate meaning of the universe. That I believed I knew. It took much reflective gazing to allow the problem to come into focus. Alright, I said, essential to the meaning in my life is the belief in the "Good news" of Jesus Christ as interpreted by St. Paul. How does that belief function? What does it contribute to make my life meaningful? Could another belief function as well?

I was excited when finally I caught the insight which opened the way to respond to those questions. I saw I had to discover what there was about me that I needed any such answer. Stock answers were saltless. By trial and error I learned how to get into myself. Silence was essential. I had to silence my voice, silence my thoughts, silence my imagination and grow still. The initial stage of understanding consists of reception, accepting, gazing, tasting, acknowledgement. I must go into myself. Poured out as I normally am, I must have a conversion to the interior, I must con-tain myself, turn inward. I warn the reader that I am describing an exercise to be practiced by himself. Without experiencing the silencing of the self, the tasting of what one experiences, one will not make sense of what follows.

What am I? What do I experience as myself? The deeper I go the clearer it becomes that I experience that I am--that I am this moment of experience. All I am, all I possess is simply and solely this momentary experiencing. Riches, status are nothing except as they enter into my moment now of experiencing, I do not have past experiences. I do not have any future experiences. I only have experience of this precise moment,

I am an event of this moment. I can prescind from all the world as I become aware I am at this moment, I am the experiencing now.

One has to be shocked with the realization that all he is and has is this experiencing moment. Once shocked he can immediately correct: there is no such thing as a moment. Every 'now' has a history and a future. It flows, flows from past, flows to future. My moment of now experiencing is a structured moment: structured by past experiences and, strangely, likewise by future needs, desires, wants. I am now experiencing as I do only because of the way past experiences have shaped me and because of the desires which move me on.[1]

There flashed to mind Nietzsche's insight that man is "will-to-power". The dynamism in that concept appealed. So I adapted the insight: I realized I am, not 'will', but 'drive' and a 'drive-to-be', not a drive-to-power. I never fully am, but I am driving to be. I am driving to express all the dimensions of my drive-to-be. Not just survival, but human expansion in freedom, intelligence, joy. Every partial expression is ordered to the expansion of the whole. Intellectual life itself is ordered to the development and expression of the whole person—indeed of the whole person within society.

This drive-to-be which I am has been structured by past experiences and moves under the attraction of desires. Summarily I see my past as a blend of the uncontrolled and the free, unfortunately with too little of the free. I am the product of so many non-chosen experiences. I had no choice coming into the world—

1. I call attention to the inadequacy of the approach I am proposing. Focusing, as it does, upon conscious experience, it can provide a significant and valuable starting point for reflection. However, it should be apparent that knowledge is not limited to immediate experience. Not only is it evident that I do not experience the event of my birth and that of my death, and yet I have no doubt the first has occurred and the second definitely will occur, but also that I remember and project by imagination and prediction. Furthermore I know who and what I am not only by experience, memory and prediction, but by scientific and philosophic understanding of what it is to be a man. This in turn involves understanding what it is to be (a man) at all. Faith likewise is a source of understanding reality, humanity, and my unique self. The basic category of understanding is not "being experienced" but "being".

no choice of parents, no choice of my body, temperament, abilities. The training at home, the schools chosen, the teachers were all decided for me. Most of the situations of growing up I submitted to or merely accepted. Years of growth were required to achieve insight into the grandeur and possibilities of freedom. Of course I have experienced the challenge and the exercise of freedom on occasions. But my life has been shaped far more by circumstances accepted than by creative experience of freedom. Insight I have but I really do not realize my unique power to make my response to events as a distinctive, free subject. It is up to me to refuse to submit to circumstances, to flee them, to change them, as well as freely to submit to them. To reach awareness of one's self as the source of free, responsible choices is the condition for full living. It takes education to freedom as well as courage to achieve such independence. But my freedom has generally been experienced as limited, limited in so many ways. Too often I have preferred to have it shackled so as to avoid the responsibility of decision.

My past experiences certainly structure my moment of experiencing but strangely so do my future wants. The very fact that it is 'now' experiencing reveals I am in time. Time implies action. So my moment of experiencing is an acting moment. My way of existing is precisely as a drive-to-be, a driving on. What drives me on, at least on the conscious level, is a want, a need, a goal, a desire. Without such I do not act, and I exist as acting. Always I am being called forward into time by wants. Hence what and how I experience at any moment is structured by my wants.

At this point I began to see why I needed an answer to the sweeping questions about life and the universe. I also came to recognize I had discovered a powerful instrument enabling me to assess any proposed answers. For I was led to list the wants, needs and desires which actually do call me on. These tell me what I have experienced as truly satisfying. I have the lived experience of the validity of these desires and their implicit value judgments. I am not able at this point to explain the need of a worldview, but it should be clear that any worldview which fails to explain the validity or value of such desires is inadequate, if not false.

As I allowed my living to unfold before me under the lens of desires I caught sight of why I was unique, yet unique as a member of the human race and of particu-

lar communities. For many of my desires I share with
all men, many I share with members of my various communities. Some are distinctive, but what chiefly charac-
terizes me as a unique person is both the ordering and
relative value I place on the different wants and the
fact that I in my individuality actually do desire them.

Time and tasting were required. Gradually the distinctive desires emerged into consciousness. Through
this lens of desires I saw the basic fact that desire
for air, food, drink drive me on, even though I rarely
attend to such wants.[2] For they are all provided for.
Yet let something hinder my breathing and it will be
evident how much I count on air. Again I am seldom conscious of any crying desire for food or drink because
they are always at hand. Not much imagination, however,
is needed to know the power of such drives. A priest
friend told me that in Japanese prison camps refined
men would squabble over one extra pea. What is important to me I ensure by habits and institutions. The
very fact of habitual provision for these needs reveals
how powerful the drive for them is. The need of shelter,
clothing, security definitely move me on, definitely influence my experiences and choices. Closely related to
such fundamental wants is the desire for peace and tran-
quility. I desire and pray for it for the world, but
I am moved to act when it is lacking around me.

It became apparent that I want things to do which
engross my attention, challenge me, and satisfy my desire to do something worthwhile. This desire means in
particular something intellectual or spiritual or needed by others. I realized I had these desires by notic-
ing the sense of wasting time when, even though necessary other tasks keep me from such work for any length
of time. Too seldom do I seek enjoyments, experiences
which evoke a genuine response of delight such as drama,
music, natural beauty, stimulating discussions, real
encounter with persons. But the need and the want are
there.

2. Sexual desires obviously constitute a special problem for a
celibate. So basic is the drive that every form of life has to
provide the means of coping with it. The profligate responds
with indulgence at will, the married person with indulgence with
his partner, but with restraint in the face of other appeals. The
celibate must freely embrace the invitation to abstinence under
the appeal of another love; he must establish tactics to lessen
the frequency and/or the power of stirrings of desire, habits of
self-control, and confidence in repentance as he struggles for
success in his commitment.

A caution: these are my desires I am reporting, desires I actually experience as appealing. Hopefully the reader will engage in a similar exercise. Then he must discover those desires which actually move him on. Honesty is crucial. He must not claim as a desire any object or any activity which he merely judges he ought to desire. If intellectual searching or love of God, for example, do not play a significant role in his life, he should not list these among his desires. For desires whose value for the individual is rooted in experience, together with the truths implicitly recognized in the experiences, are what enable the individual to test competing world-views.

Let me go on. I desire love, friends. I need the experience of encountering another, of delight in the presence of another, the sense of easy familiarity. Not only am I aware of such desire in the delight experienced, but also in the loneliness felt when it is absent.

I want to love God, to experience His presence, to pray, to worship. If such experiences are absent for too long I genuinely miss them and feel a drive to recapture that sense of presence. Indeed I feel shallow without it. I want to offer Mass and function as a priest.

I want to be free, to shape my own life, to make my decisions. I very much want to know, to understand. I want to understand myself, the meaning of life, what is happening to me and to society. I want some part in developing this universe in terms of scientific understanding, technological control and sociological-political structuring. I want all these developments to contribute to the elimination of human suffering and economic deprivation. I want men to enjoy peace, everywhere, freedom and happiness.

I want to keep on living, indeed forever. It is not that I often think consciously about eternal life, but I do feel the desire when I reflect on death and see death as the gateway to life. While I rarely attend to the afterlife with its rewards or punishments, I think it forms an unconscious assumption--much as the desire for air--and if I were seriously to doubt it I might well feel desperate.

It took days for these facts about myself to emerge and take shape. I found a new sense of identity and security as I grew to know myself. I felt no one could challenge what I knew from within. Limited as was this area of knowledge it gave me roots in experience rather than theory for guiding my life and for assessing any worldview. But I soon realized how very significant in this understanding of myself was the order in my desires.

I expand in time one act at a time and one desire at a time: at least one prime, ordering desire. Multiple wants may, of course, be fulfilled by one act, but if so, they have coalesced under one characterizing goal. It is next to impossible to explain why the different desires arise. They are so many and the causes for their emergence and dominance at any particular moment are often incalculable. In fact they frequently appear to be unordered and of quasi-equal strength of appeal. Actually a commanding order of priority operates among one's desires. Let the most appealing object engross one's attention, the appeal will cease immediately if breathing is endangered. Beauty can scarcely attract if survival is challenged or hunger experienced. And the measure of the priority is not consciousness of pleasure or a sense of the importance. Rooted in one's deepest self lies the ordering of these basic needs.

We have no control over the ordering of desires according to basic needs. But we become who we are through the ordering and priority of our other desires. Is physical activity sacrificed to intellectual activity or the reverse? Is present sensual pleasure sacrificed to future professional achievement? How different is the man with family as his main concern from one who places sexual gratification as his. In the former instance does love of wife or love of children hold first place?

As I became accustomed to experiencing myself as this drive-to-be moved on by desires the two essential, constitutive elements of a meaningful life took shape as inevitable. For I found myself coming back again and again to two key questions. How do I harmonize my desires? How do these multiple desires and needs blend into a harmonious constellation so that I am truly one? Whenever light seemed to illumine this problem, explaining why I acted, I would be shocked by a deeper question. Suppose you succeed in harmonizing your desires so that one definite desire moves you on, explaining why you act as you do, is there any sense to acting at all? Does the blending of desires presuppose

that the whole makes sense? Is there any meaning overarching the entire series of acts which make up my life?

These two questions fought for attention, each
claiming priority. And both claims were valid. Harmonization of desires clearly held psychological priority. Overarching meaning was logically prior. Finally,
probably because I was at peace in the harmonization of
my desires, I opted to pursue first the question of overarching meaning.

The problem shows its head this way. As a drive-
to-be I am moved on by desires. The countless needs
and desires emerge and call me unto action. I respond
to the appeal or the compulsion. Does that suffice to
explain why I act? If I am harmonized in my desires,
would that explain the meaning in my life? Or does the
whole series of acts need a justification, a meaning as
well?

It was the plot of a mystery story which provided
the clue to the insight I needed. I had read John Le
Carre's The Spy Who Came In From the Cold, years earlier,
and now the plot took on new significance. The conduct
of Leamas, the principal character, I recalled, might be
interpreted by an outsider as merely a series of acts
aptly explained by the immediate inclinations and situation. But they were linked together by Leamas's intention and had a very different meaning. Beyond Leamas'
intention, however, the same acts had a totally different meaning for he was being used by Control.

Let me limn the plot. The characters who inter-
ested me are Leamas, who retires from chief of British
intelligence in Berlin, Control (no other name is given),
head of the entire British intelligence system, Liz, a
girl with whom Leamas unwillingly becomes involved,
Mundt, chief of Communist operations in Berlin, Leamas's
counterpart, and Fiedler, assistant to Mundt.

Leamas had grown to hate his counterpart, Mundt,
because regularly at crucial points Mundt has succeeded
in thwarting his plots and, as the story opens, has just
killed the last of his agents. In his interview with
Control upon retiring this attitude is brought into the
open. Control invites him to engage in a subtle plot
to destroy Mundt. Instead of a normal retirement,
Leamas takes a serious demotion to a lowly sort of
clerk's job. He drinks heavily, lets his resentment be
known until he is fired. To survive he takes a job re-
turning books in a library where he meets Liz, a librar-

ian and part-time Communist. In his loneliness he becomes involved with her, regretting it, for aware of
what he is doing, he does not want anyone else hurt.
One day he belligerently creates a scene at the butcher
shop, throws a few punches, gets arrested and is given
a few months in prison. Really down and out he is approached upon his release by agents of Fiedler. He
seems ripe for exploitation of his secret information.
Bitter at the treatment he has received after years of
dangerous service, financially destitute, practically a
drunken bum, he is ready to forget patriotic loyalty
and to trade his knowledge for money. Spirited off by
the agents he is brought to East Germany where Fiedler
interrogates him for weeks.

Now he is in the position Control and he had gamb-
led on. Fiedler, a devoted communist, has become suspicious of Mundt's loyalty. Leamas proceeds to reveal
a secret operation which had sent him to different cit-
ies in Europe to deposit large sums in banks under a
certain name. The details are calculated to allow Fiedler to link such deposits with trips by Mundt to the
same places, soon followed by British successes in
thwarting Communist plots. In this way Fiedler builds
so strong a case against Mundt that he files charges
against him as a British agent.

At the trial Leamas repeats his story and the evidence mounts convincingly. However Liz suddenly is
introduced to the court and questioning reveals that
shortly after Leamas disappeared men recognizable as
agents for Control visited her and provided substantial
funds for her support. It now becomes apparent that
Leamas' conduct and story are an elaborate plot by Control to discredit Mundt. Consequently Mundt is vindi-
cated and Fiedler is removed from office.

An uninformed observer would interpret Leamas'
behavior as simply a series of actions fulfilling multiple needs. He was disappointed so he drank; as he
drank he became unreliable, so he lost his job. And so
through the chain of events there was no meaning beyond
the succession of choices.

On the other hand the reader knows that behind the
apparent succession of acts is an overarching meaning
since Leamas is using these ploys to destroy Mundt.
Beyond Leamas' governing intention, however, is Control's
meaning, for the goal of Control is not to destroy Mundt
since he really is a British agent, but to protect him
by destroying Fiedler, who has become suspicious of him.

Leamas, incidentally, is a very disillusioned man when he realizes how he has been duped by Control and bitter at the brutal use of innocent Liz, who is to be killed escaping rather than to remain available to be used later against Mundt. He, Leamas, dies also.

This detailed illustration poses the issue. I am this moment of experience. Being in time I am by acting. I act under the attraction of wants. I am drawn by one desire after another. Am I, is my life, sufficiently explained by this succession of wants drawing me on? Or is there some pattern which binds this succession together in an overarching meaning? Must I to some extent operate with some overarching meaning? If I do not understand any such, must I presuppose there is such?

It is important that the point of the illustration from LeCarre be grasped. The meaning imparted by Control to the succession of events is what must be realized. The series of events possessed an objective ordering not only beyond what an uninformed observer would perceive, but even beyond what Leamas intended. Instead of being a succession of unordered events, each motivated by the obvious immediate desire and influenced by the obvious immediate circumstances, they actually were ordered to the protection of Mundt and the removal of Fiedler. Are my actions ordered to some goal, according to some pattern, beyond the obvious response to the desires which prompt the actions? Do they together with nature and all other human actions build toward anything? The answer can be negative or positive. If positive, the answer can be simply that there is some such ordering or one may posit some specific explanation of the ordering such as Communism or Christian theistic humanism. In the latter cases one does not assume to be able to identify the particular contribution of every event. Yet there is assurance that they do contribute somehow and with a definite orientation.

The question of an overarching meaning does not arise early in life or indeed often. As the person grows he is lured on by wants. Achievement of immediate goals, satisfaction of immediate desires generally suffice. Yet, this is so, I believe, because one assumes things are ordered and that the whole has meaning. In Berger's Rumor of Angels one of the 'signals of transcendence' is order. The mother calms the frightened child by cuddling and reassuring him--"everything is alright". Many indeed seem to live without raising the question of the meaning of the whole, finding the

succession of wants adequate. This is particularly the
case of a person with health, an engrossing occupation,
satisfying social relations and financial success. I
submit this works only because implicitly meaning for
the whole is assumed, and one keeps busy pursuing goal
after immediate goal. It may also demand avoiding the
theatre or music. Artists lift the veil on inadequate
lives and the successful business man, for example, may
have difficulty avoiding further questioning if he at-
tends plays by Tennessee Williams or Edward Albee, not
to mention Sartre or Beckett.

About twelve years ago I ran into the attitude
among some students in a course on the philosophy of
religion that the question of God simply did not arise
for them. Their lives were satisfying and if they were
forced to face the question of God and afterlife, it
simply meant: if there is a God and there is an afterlife, great. It will be a delightful surprise to discover this is so. But they did not need God now nor experience any question about God.

These students were, I believe, riding the crest
of secularization. Almost immediately afterwards, the
counterculture surfaced and what had seemed to render
lives satisfying no longer had any meaning for many
young people. The structures of society which had ab-
sorbed the interests of previous students no longer
made sense.

For if society's concrete goals are embraced, the
procedures and stages to achieve them will be accepted
and make sense. But if the goals do not appeal or make
sense, then procedures will be senseless, unless they
happen to appeal in themselves. Material achievements
in terms of accumulation of wealth and status symbols
warranted postponement of enjoyment, remote preparation
and hard work. Many in the counter culture rejected
such goals and so found the demands senseless.

Such a train of reflection led me to see how
strange was my question. None of us lives by theoretical insights but by customs, life-styles that satisfy.
Never before had I asked--is there an overarching meaning in life? Like everyone else I had not learned my
most important truths and values theoretically, but by
living. Then why was I asking it? I realized, as I
have said, that I was in a privileged position: from
within the experience of meaning being reborn I could
perceive the articulation of a meaningful life. Not
only was I driven by the desire to understand but by

the desire to help others. The present train of thought
penetrated me with the light that understanding would
not bestow or restore meaning to others in need. Indeed
few would be drawn to entertain my question or follow my
reflections to get my answers. And still, I thought,
they might. While it is true we live by life-styles,
how do we handle unhappiness or conflict? It is at this
point that reflective, theoretical understanding really
can help. If I could succeed in understanding the functioning of these elements in meaning, others confused
or unhappy might understand what was happening to them
and discover for themselves how to incarnate these elements in their own life-style.

Encouraged that my efforts to understand were of
value I pushed on. I am a drive-to-be drawn on by desires. Some things may appeal only because of their relation to something else which does exert intrinsic
appeal. But not only must I experience the intrinsic
appeal in certain desires but the whole succession of
wants and desires must have meaning and appeal as well.
If the whole succession of wants does not have or is
not assumed to have meaning and appeal none will. The
meaning and appeal of seeking health, education, wealth,
success presupposes that living has meaning. If being
alive is meaningless, then so are all the activities
which make up one's life. The succession, as a whole,
of actions which constitute life must 'make sense' to
the mind for the person to want to live.

Most of us 'feel' rather than think our way
through life. Yet every human person has to answer for
himself at least implicitly the question: is there an
overarching meaning to life? To 'feel' is to answer
implicitly. But if the question raises its head expli-
citly, the person has a powerful instrument for confidently facing the challenge if he has gone through the
process described and become conscious of his actually
experienced desires and values. He can assess any possible answer. Any position which denies or fails to
explain what he has experienced as true and satisfying
must be wrong or at least inadequate.

When I found myself facing the basic question,
"Is there any overarching meaning?" I knew I could
leap positively and strongly beyond this. Yet I deliberately paused for not too long before I would have
hesitated and I sensed many would just as strongly answer 'no'. Those for whom life is absurd profess, ex-
plicitly or implicitly, that there is no overarching
meaning. No wonder life is experienced as painful. No

wonder the attidue is--'I didn't ask to be born'. No
wonder suicide is the only serious question. So long
as one has the vitality, the opportunity to indulge
one's pleasures, one may ignore the absurdity of it all.
The nihilism of existentialist despair which sees the
total enterprise of life and universe as absurd is post-
Christian. And it emerged after technology so liberated
men from urgent needs that in the leisure and power provided men could ask what should civilization set its
aim upon. What is life's purpose? Since God and religion
were dead for so many and since calculative thinking
dominated reasoning the answer was inescapable - none.

I weighed this answer. My own experience of joy
in life, joy in loving, joy in being made me unsympa-
thetic to this existentialist despair. Besides my experience of joy, however, was the conviction that in
limited areas of life there definitely was meaning.
The implicit value judgments in these joyful experiences, which I knew were true, the recognition. of ration-
al meaning in speech, and the clear rationality of so
many limited areas of life told me that the whole must
also have meaning and that existentialist despair was
wrong. There has to be some overarching meaning, but
what is it?

Is there an overarching meaning? What is it? I
saw these were two non-questions for me. I was definitely committed to Christ; his "Good News" as interpreted
by St. Paul gave rich meaning to the entire creation.
Then I was jolted. If I am on the level of meaning I
had to face the reality of an entire spectrum of worldviews which actually function to provide this element
of a meaningful life, the overarching meaning. People
lived intensely meaningful lives who did not embrace
Christianity. Within my experience competing for men's
allegiance and seeking to discover perspectives immediately related to contemporary experience are Communism,
scientific humanism, Christian theistic humanism, and
various efforts of the counter-culture or forms of
Eastern religions. Most people in the West seem to me
to embrace one or other or a combination of these worldviews. I am not attempting to investigate how a person
acquires whatever overarching meaning he may have and
certainly I am not claiming one has to establish it or
even the need of any such reflectively. Most people
grow up into or assume one of these worldviews. They
absorb it with their community lifestyle. In fact we
are all quite capable of living with contradictions
within our views. The professed Christian for example,

36

who absorbs from his culture the belief that only common sense experience and the natural sciences warrant truth is living an unconscious contradiction. Many of his basic tenets cannot be so warranted. Their justification relies on religious experience or faith or philosophic understanding.

I began to see that I had to change the second question to "What is the overarching meaning for me?" I also began to see the limits of the method I had discovered. Becoming aware of what really counts in my life will indeed enable me to assess any worldview. This in principle makes it possible to test these competing overarching meanings measuring their adequacy in explaining the multiple desires I have experienced as valid values. The test may well suffice psychologically without logically sufficing to confirm the truth of my overarching meaning. Christian theistic humanism alone is adequate for my constellation of wants and desires. Commitment to this belief brings great satisfaction. But the implicit tenets, the reality of God, the divinity of Christ, the veracity of scripture and so forth demand independent and proper verification. Otherwise we may be operating on a basis of wish fulfillment. Meaning in life, I now realized, refers to an attitude of consciousness, not to objective truth. Obviously meaning may be found along with error. Theists and atheists both may experience meaning in their lives. Yet the assertions implicit in the two life-styles are contradictory and cannot both be true. This attitude of consciousness, it is clear, consists primarily in belief or conviction that one has the truth.

The lineaments of meaning were beginning to stand out more sharply. I now saw that recapturing belief in the "Good News" of Jesus Christ in St. Paul's interpretation contributed to the rebirth of meaning in my life not because it was true but because my believing it was true provided an overarching meaning to life. That was how it functioned. If I had lost faith in Christ completely and embraced scientific humanism I would have rebuilt meaning anyway. So long as a person believed there was some overarching meaning this would suffice for a meaningful life. Most people assent to an overarching meaning not in any explicit way but by embracing the worldview of a community life-style.

This was beginning to look like sheer relativism. Doesn't it make any difference which worldview one embraces? Doesn't truth matter? That such a question could emerge forced me to turn back and look again at my method. I had overstated the case. Truth is involved. What one accepts as true profoundly affects the kind of person, the kind of society which will result. Belief in error will hurt person and society. Furthermore my experienced desires and values do operate to exclude as false worldviews which deny my implicit value judgments or which would render them theoretically impossible. They exclude as inadequate a worldview unable to allow for or explain them. In fact I found that the experience of evaluating the competing worldviews by reference to experienced desires and values proved so psychologically satisfying that one could mistakenly think one had positively proved the truth of the overarching meaning which satisfies. For many it would suffice. Logically however the basic implicit affirmations embodied in the worldview require positive verification.

This line of questioning aided by a story I recalled led me to enter into an exercise of testing the competing worldviews in the light of my list of desires. It seems a Rabbi Eisik of Cracow had a strange dream directing him to go to Prague. There, under a certain bridge, he would discover a treasure. He could ignore the dream the first and second times, but when the same dream recurred on the third successive night he knew he had to go. He located the bridge alright but feared to dig lest the guards on patrol arrest him. In his fear he blurted out the story of his dreams when his loitering prompted a guard to question him. The guard burst into laughter, "You actually believed this dream and wasted time and energy to come here? I'd never be so silly. Why I had a dream that I would find a treasure if I'd go to Cracow to the home of some Rabbi Eisik. In a corner behind the stove I'd find it. But I am too reasonable to waste my time following dreams." The Rabbi thanked him, hastened home and found the treasure in his own home.[3] So often what we seeek we already possess, but strangers make us see it. As I brought the competing worldviews to judgment before my experienced desires and values I learned two things. No viable worldview lacks important values and truths. And every worldview humiliates me by the greater esteem each has for some truth or value I profess. Indeed I do discover from these strangers what I actually possessed without properly appreciating it.

3. M. Eliade, <u>Myths, Dreams and Mysteries</u>, New York: Harper & Brothers, 1960, p. 244.

The communist's concern for human suffering and injustice, for instance, their determined efforts to solve these problems shame me. Some years ago in a French communist-Christian dialogue, a communist challenged: We don't want to hear about Christ. Tell us where the Christians are. I must strike my breast in repentance. Their commitment to the poor and the powerless drives me back to Christ's challenge:

> *"Come. You have my Father's blessing! Inherit the*
> *kingdom prepared for you from the creation of the*
> *world. For I was hungry and you gave me food, I was*
> *thirsty and you gave me drink. I was a stranger and*
> *you welcomed me, naked and you clothed me...as often*
> *as you did it for one of my least brothers, you did*
> *it for me." (Mt. 25, 34).*

This identification of Christ with men Paul proclaims in his teaching of the mystical body of Christ. It forms the framework and the motivation of Pope John XXIII's encyclical Mother and Teacher, which prescribes that the imbalances in the different sectors of our economy, national and international, must be corrected. The Second Vatican Council's exciting Pastoral Constitution of the Church in the Modern World sets the Church positively in the stance of sharing all human concerns and insists on the obligation to humanize our social institutions. More recent developments in the Church on national and international levels confirm the Church's intention to keep this stance.

Communism, I found, awakens me to the importance of these values in my own tradition. Yet at the same time I recognize it as destructive of human freedom. Not only do I have the witness of numerous men who embraced Communism in noble selflessness only to leave because their freedom was stifled[4] but I see creative liberty in principle menaced by subjection to a controlling group's non-absolute, arbitrary judgments. Communism aims at a collectivity of individuals rather than a society of free subjects.

Scientific humanism, on the other hand, insists on individual freedom. So much appeals to me in this

4. R. Crossman, ed., The God That Failed, (by Andre Gide, Richard Wright, Ignazio Silone, Stephen Spendar, Arthur Koestler, Louis Fischer), N.Y.: Bantam Books, 1952. Gulag Archipelago by A. Solzhenitzin as well as his other works eloquently testifies to the same.

world-view. I imagine a profound sense of liberation
would pervade the person embracing it--at least initially. One exalts in the liberty and power to decide what
to do with one's life and what is to constitute value.
The goal of humanizing this universe: developing the
sciences and technology to control the earth, devising
institutions to benefit all man--such a goal is really
ennobling and engrossing.

Sharing Communism's determination to develop this
universe and eliminate injustice, but without the obvious shackling of freedom, this world-view likewise
drove me back to reexamine my Christian heritage. This
time Paul leapt to mind. God's plan is to restore all
things in Jesus Christ. (Eph. 1, 10). The whole of
creation groans in anticipation of redemption. In the
primitive covenant of man with God, God entrusted to
him the task of developing this universe. (Gen. 1,
28). With Christ man retains that assigned task but
fulfills it in and through and with Christ.

Personal development and fulfillment is impossible
without Christ. The weakness of man born from Adam
cries for relief in the experience of the conflict of
the two laws within him. "What a wretched man I am!
Who can free me from this body under the power of death?
All praise to God, through Jesus Christ our Lord!"
(Rom. 7, 24). In Christ we are free: "The Lord is the
Spirit, and where the Spirit of the Lord is, there is
freedom." (2 Cor. 3, 17). "Therefore...we are not
children of a slave girl but of a mother who is free.
It was for liberty that Christ freed us." (Gal. 4, 31).
Indeed "my brothers, remember that you have been called
to live in freedom..." (Gal. 5, 13).

In this freedom we retain the original task to
develop this universe, now to be restored in Jesus
Christ. Thus instead of humanizing the universe we are
called to Christmanize it. Facing the same tasks as
the scientific humanists we humbly cooperate and prof-
fer the message, the life, the power of Jesus Christ to
accomplish them. The message constitutes us transcen-
dental critics of every form of life: do these structures reveal the esteem for each human person with whom
Christ identifies himself? Any practice, any institution which hurts a human person is to that extent not
Christian. But beyond a message the Christian carries
the life and power of the new life of Christ to effect
what is envisioned.

So appealing has been the vision of scientific

humanism that many Christians have embraced it in a
process of secularization. What is needed, I sensed,
is rather the sacralizing of the secular. Let the life-
style center upon human development: means of survival,
education, cultural development, expansion of freedom,
experience of enjoying what we do, the spread of love,
discovery of social structures which allow the individual to become himself, discovery of the mysteries of
nature and life so man can grow and control and humanize the universe. And with such commitment can grow
the recognition of the need of the new life and power
Christ brings to accomplish all this. I caught the
insight that such prior commitment could measure the
need of expressions of religion, such as prayer, pro-
clamation of scripture, sacrifice: as much as is
needed to enable us to live as Christmen and to fulfill
our destiny to Christmanize the universe. And the measure of the kind and amount of religious institution will
be the need to provide the channels for prayer, scripture, sacrament and sacrifice. It was not naturalistic
humanism I was proposing but the realization that human
fulfillment is impossible without Christ.

Scientific humanism certainly helped me appreciate
my own tradition. Its emphases evidence genuine values.
But as an overarching meaning itself, I find scientific
humanism a position for the young, healthy and intelligent. While its enthusiastic drive for scientific development, healthy living, enjoyment can harmonize
one's energies, what does it offer the sick and suffering or the old? Or does one cease to count in these
circumstances? The sick and the old can hardly drive
for the development of this universe. Is there, then,
no overarching meaning for them?

The spread of the mentality proper to scientific
humanism I likewise saw as destructive of the human
person and of society. More and more it pervades our
culture with the conviction that the only way to warrant any position is common sense or the natural sciences, and that man's role is to control all aspects of
universe and life. Not only has this mentality developed the present technocracy so crippling to the human
person, but it is corroding all ethical values. Science can study partial views of what is and people's
opinions. It cannot deal with the whole nor with what
should be. Ethics is intelligent reflection on what
fulfills man as a whole. Omission of the ethical dimension, of the dimension of rights, which science must
omit, is behind the widespread acceptance of birth-
control, behind the speculation favoring genetic con-

41

trol with the government to determine who may have
children, behind the movement toward the licensed killing of the old, the sick, the retarded, which may well
lead to killing of political opponents. My desire for
freedom, my love of men, my desire for truth warn me
against scientific humanism. But I had further reasons
for rejecting communism and scientific humanism.

I must hasten to insist that we all seem able to
live unconscious of contradictions within our beliefs
and convictions. Many scientific humanists live with
such integrity and uprightness that I would entrust my
property and life to them more confidently than to many
Christians. Many of them so esteem the values of love
and life that they would be the last to subscribe to
such evils as I have mentioned. I refer, not to scientific humanists, the persons, but to the principles of
scientific humanism, which indeed, I believe, permit
such conclusions as I have listed and which indeed have
already been proposed.

But I had further reasons for rejecting communism
and scientific humanism. For myself, as for all those
who have experienced the living presence of God, worldviews such as these simply cannot stand. They deny my
experienced encounter with God, my experienced sense of
satisfaction, which belief in God provides in the face
of chance, death and suffering. They fail to make
sense of the numerous people I esteem who profess shared
experience of God and whose lives give such impressive
testimony to their belief. History parades billions of
believers including the most brilliant thinkers through
the ages. Atheistic positions face a serious challenge
to explain these facts away.[5]

5. I do not offer these remarks by way of proof. They may serve
to dispose a person to face a serious examination of the question
of God's existence. While I do not intend to propose any proofs
I would like to observe that in years of teaching proofs of God's
existence, I have realized that unless one encounters God in experience one will not accept any proof. For proofs simply cannot
lead one to 'know' God, but only 'to know about' Him. The function of any attempted argument is to justify the theistic interpretation of one's subjective experience. Supposing one has experienced God, reasoning enters to show that the interpretation
that it is God one has encountered is sound. While no proof can
lead an unbeliever to experience God, it may eliminate intellectual barriers to this experience or its theistic interpretation.
Failure to recognize how proofs function, just where they fit,
has contributed to the rejection of traditional proofs and to an
attitude of fideism.

Any overarching meaning which denies the reality
of God not only denies my experienced encounter of God,
it also cannot square with my desire for love. In loving another one experiences something absolute and eternal. This is the case in heightened moments of union,
but also in moments of sacrifice, even for a stranger.
There is almost a sense of a 'beyond' which is absolute
and eternal. Christian theistic humanism lets me realize that in this experience of human love my love opens
into love of God. For indeed the loved one is lovable
because God created him as an expression of God Himself.
In love, then, one meets God. The risk in loving is
grounded: the inherent tragedy in every human love
seemingly ended by death is transformed by belief that
the beloved lives and that the love will continue for
eternity. The danger of loving unwisely too is protected against for one knows that the person is worth
loving anyway, for he indeed does reflect the goodness
of God, and one surrenders in love because God invites
one to love. Without risk love is impossible. Christian theistic humanism encourages and grounds prudent
risk.

Most people, I realized, never think about love in
this framework. Indeed many who do not profess belief
in God love deeply. I submit that in their love they
meet God unknowingly and implicitly affirm His being.[6]

On the other hand those who raise the question of
God's existence and deny it cannot consistently love at
all.[7] This sense of the absolute and the eternal experienced in loving ought logically to be acknowledged
by them to be illusory. If the person is consistent,
he will eliminate that dimension and focus upon himself.
Rather than offering himself to the other--even at the
price of sacrifice and death--he should logically treat
love as a delightful titillation to be indulged in so
long as it satisfies. Why risk the pain of betrayal or
that of separation by death? Atheists do love, I am

6. One of the problems many young people are experiencing is a
seeming lack of experience of God. They do not seem to encounter
God in liturgy. God meets them rather in love, in service and in
sacrifice. But because the implication of such experiences have
not been worked out they do not recognize that they have met God.

7. Sartre is strikingly consistent in believing neither in God
nor in love. I owe this insight to Richard Cobb-Stevens of Boston
College.

sure, but only by ignoring the contradiction between what they experience and what they profess. Implicit truths work themselves out I mused, and atheism, given time, will work itself out to the prevention of love and the destruction of the human person.[8]

Much more thought and study went into this assessment of communism and scientific humanism than I have time to recount. Perhaps, however, I have sufficiently illustrated how I tested competing worldviews by means of my experienced desires and values. Many will not share my desire for God and immortality nor reflect on the implications of love from my perspective. Their experienced desires may differ from mine as well as their understanding of these worldviews. If they truly become aware of the desires which move them on, which count in their lives, they will experience the same

8. At this point I muse about the similarity of criticism by conflicting world-views. To the atheist the Christian theist is deluded, fails to recognize the contradictions within his system, covers up the evils which have resulted from religions, indeed is blind to the harm to the human person inherent in religious belief. On the other hand I am puzzled how an atheistic position can successfully operate to provide an overarching meaning. Not only do I fault it as inadequate to the needs and drives of man, not only do I consider it makes love impossible and so is destructive of the human person, not only do I agree with Jung that only religious encounter with an absolute can provide the strength for the individual to withstand the pressure of socialization; but I find a basic intellectual contradiction in the very formulation of the position.

To intimate the basic intellectual contradiction I find in the very formulation of the atheistic position I shall use an approach found in Longeran's Insight. Being may be defined as that which is open to intelligent inquiry and reasonable affirmation. Proportionate being is that which is open to intelligent inquiry, reasonable affirmation and sensible experience. Naturalism maintains that proportionate being is all there is. Every form of atheism is a form of naturalism. Naturalism reasons that every explanation demands that the ultimate be accepted as mere matter of fact. What then is the ultimate explanation of the universe? Proportionate being is mere matter of fact. But mere matter of fact is precisely that which is not open to intelligent inquiry and reasonable affirmation. Therefore it is not being. Outside of being there is nothing. Naturalism therefore proposes that the ultimate in explaining the universe is nothing.

The skeletal criticism of atheistic world views will satisfy no one, but does provide an outline of my evaluation of them. I can only explain their effectiveness in providing overarching meaning to people's lives by suggesting that atheists inconsistently affirm an absolute and especially in loving ignore or suspend the contraction.

confidence I experienced in testing these views. Meaning, I emphasize again, refers not directly to truth
but to an attitude of consciousness.

Of the two remaining 'isms' I sensed were competing in the West as worldviews I recognized I knew little
about the Eastern religions. Their contemplative appeal I already possessed in my life and somehow I
sensed they would not satisfy my desire for man's development and control of the universe. I spent little
time examining these as an overarching meaning.

I was, however, much attracted by the counter culture. As I saw the movement there was almost violent
reaction against technocratic structuring of life with
a counter emphasis on feeling, freedom and enjoyment.
I agreed that excessive socratic living had set us on
the way to the death of man. It was not God's death,
but man's we were sensing. To preserve life the new
consciousness released the dionysian and appollonian
elements in man.[9] Instead of planned living, there
would be spontaneity. Instead of postponed living,
there would be 'now' living. Instead of cerebral control, feeling would decide. Instead of discipline and
restraint, freedom. Whatever one does or believes must
be linked with felt need or satisfaction.

I saw so much I could learn from this way of life.
I am much too cerebral and I have so often failed to
experience the present through concern about past or
future. I want to take my stance in the present and to
ensure that I want to do whatever I am doing. This
stance, I saw, could liberate me from the cult of the
past. Eager about present living and needs I could measure the value of past thought and achievement by their
contribution to what the present needs demanded. I felt
this new consciousness provided a prism for reexamining
my entire Christian tradition.

9. As I read Nietzche's Birth of Tragedy there are the three elements in man: the dionysian, the apollonian and the socratic. The
pulsating, dynamic thrust to life and communion is the dionysian
element which cannot be expressed without some form. The apollonian element is the creative imagination which provides this concrete from of expression of the dionysian. The socratic, in principle, allows for conceptualization and assessment of the suitabil-
ity and validity of the expression. Excessive development of the
socratic element of man led to repression especially of the dionysian, but also of the apollonian. Thus was structured technocratic society and thus was triggered the revolt of the counter culture which released the dionysian and apollonian elements.

As a total view, however, it is woefully inadequate. Valuable as it is as a corrective, its focus on feeling without guidance of thought makes it destructive of the person. I do not see how love is possible when immediate satisfaction warrants decisions. Its excessive focus on immediate pleasure impedes the requisite training and planning required by developed societies. In fact the counter-culture is parasitic upon establishment culture which provides the necessities.

These days had brought me alive as never before. The thrilling sense that all I am is caught up in this moment of experiencing, this dynamic driving-to-be, had been confirmed by accepting the stance in the present of the NOW generation. Everything remained to be done and all I am to be is constantly at issue in my free choices. I found myself running my beliefs through the prism of this new stance and discovered a profound reordering resulted. Perhaps I was able to risk such radical gazing because my confidence had become rooted in the consciousness of desires and values experienced as really counting in my life and the honest facing of competing worldviews. I learned so much about my own values from sympathetic but testing study of these other ways of life.

The radical questioning took the form of asking am I primarily a Catholic, a Christian or a member of the family of man? I discovered the answer is none of these. I discovered my overarching meaning is a person, Jesus Christ. I give myself primarily to Jesus Christ. But Jesus Christ is but a medium by which I go to the Blessed Trinity. Once united in this unique way to the Blessed Trinity, I do not turn back, but somehow pass through the Blessed Trinity to the family of man. God's love, his concern, his plan is primarily for the entire family of man, for man's control and development of the universe, for the happiness of all. I share in all of man's needs, challenges, successes, joys. Indeed I join every man, communist, scientific humanist, Jew, Moslem, fellow Christian in the labor of humanizing this universe. In awe I realize that the Blessed Trinity is living through me, needs me to experience human problems in my unique way. All of human life from birth to death, the life of everyone from laborer to industrialist, to politician, to statesman, to social engineer is important, for the Blessed Trinity lives through men. God has inserted the new life and power of Jesus Christ, the medium through which they engage in life's work, into the world so that the goal is to Christmanize, rather than humanize, the universe. My ultimate objective then is not to become united to God, but to allow God to live and work through me. Whatever furthers man's control of the universe, whatever expands man's freedom, power, joy, whatever helps society become a loving union of equals is in the direction of Christmanizing.[10]

This is the view of Christian theistic humanism which now operated as overarching meaning in my life. It makes life an adventure from childhood to death. I am so impressed that challenge to growth should never cease. Every situation in every stage of my life I am called to let the Blessed Trinity experience it through me. The whole of my life indeed has meaning. The desires, distinctively mine, obviously are grounded. Union with God in love not only satisfies my desire to love God but is the very means of turning me out to love others. Like God my entire life is to love. Prayer, worship are needed to keep alive and growing the union with God as well as to allow my choices to be indeed what the Blessed Trinity wants. My role of priest stands as most important in its function to communicate and nurture this new life and power in Jesus Christ. Not only do I feel called to freedom but this power of love is great enough to effect the harmony of desires productive of true interior liberty. All the human desires for knowledge and developing this universe are transformed in the goal of Christmanizing all. Death has been conquered becoming the gateway to life eternal.

No one can deny my experienced sense of satisfaction in this overarching meaning. One may be able to

10. It is extremely difficult to express this relationship. God the Blessed Trinity, is immutable, infinite, possessing all being and perfection in a transcendent, eminent manner. Nothing can be added to God. And yet, in some mysterious way, without the Incarnation of the Second Person of the Blessed Trinity, God would not have the human mode of experiencing. Analogously, without me, God would not have the distinctive, unique mode of experiencing which I am and which I remain when united through Jesus Christ to the Blessed Trinity. Thus God does not experience in any strict sense. But since God dwells creatively within me He too is the source of every action I perform. My actions are distinctive and unique. Therefore God posits actions through me which in their uniqueness He could not posit without me.

United in the Blessed Trinity I go to the family of man. This very union gives the richest explanation of ecumenism. But I need the Catholic Church as the community which gives me Christ.

challenge my consistency or more fundamentally the truth of the implicit affirmations in this Christian humanism. But I am concerned with meaning not with truth, even though I do indeed believe what I have said is true.

At this point I felt I understood how the overarching meaning functioned as an essential constitutent in a meaningful life. In fact I was tempted to rush ahead to test my analysis by examining how pain affected my overarching meaning to bring about my non-meaningful mood. I resisted the impulse for I still had the second essential constituent to explain. Psychologically the harmonization of desires is even prior to the question of the overarching meaning. There can be little meaning in life unless I am somehow one. How do I blend my multiple desires into a harmonious constellation?

CHAPTER FOUR

Harmonization: Subordinating/Dominant Desire

A rhythm blending the enthusiastic and the routine governs most lives. Times of fervor, times of quiet habits. In the rebirth of meaning I had experienced a sense that Christ called me, wanted me, had something for me to do. This fused me and gave me joy. I tried to live out the belief that the Blessed Trinity experienced human life through me. I am this drive-to-be led on by desires and what I had to do was let the Blessed Trinity experience these situations, these choices, these acts through me. This affected everything. I even drove a car differently. Relating to other drivers, kind or mean, I tried to react toward them as the Blessed Trinity desired--with love.

In this time of enthusiasm the overarching meaning seemed enough. I just wanted to live out this new way of life. No need of further reflection. But I soon remembered that times of fervor pass and I would need sober understanding of what was happening. I faced the fact that I still had no answer to the second basic question. I still did not understand how my desires had been so harmonized. Indeed why did this sense of being called, this sense of being a needed and unique instrument of the Blessed Trinity to bring their love to the world fuse me into a whole? I had much to do.

I mused myself back to the neutral, phenomenal description of myself as this moment of experiencing, this drive-to-be structured by my desires. At this point I understood that the succession of desires as a whole needed and had meaning. More significant than the actual desires experienced is the constellation into which they are ordered. It seemed obvious that they had to be harmonized but I found myself asking why must they?

It took hours of gazing, probing, asking before the truth took shape. I can act only if I am. I can be only if I am one. I can act with meaning and desire only if I am meaningful to myself. I can be meaningful to myself only if I am consciously one. I can be consciously one only if in my desires I am harmonized as one under one definite controlling desire.

This felt so true, so satisfying that I thought that it was the best thing I had ever written and that it had brought me to the verge of complete insight. The self consciously identifies itself because one desire harmonizes all the rest. But how does this one definite desire exercise its control to harmonize the other desires?

For a long time all I could see was that somehow a person is whole, is one in all he does. What kept me from catching the needed insight was the complexity of the constellation of desires and the fact, which I finally grasped, that the controlling desire can function in two ways. It can harmonize by subordinating all other desires under itself or by being dominant among autonomous desires.

Under stress I operate under a subordinating desire, but only for a time. Anyone who has really wanted something so badly that he sacrifices convenience and other satisfactions to get it knows how a subordinating desire functions. The student who pushes himself for an examination by going into isolation, working without sleep or food is operating under a subordinating desire. I cannot live long with such stress. I follow my various desires unless they interfere with my dominant desire. The latter functions as a negative norm. The man who enjoys his work, indulges in golf and parties unless they jeopardize his primary goal is operating under a dominant desire.

I knew I was not one of those few men strong enough to live harmonized under one subordinating desire. Apart from rare periods or situations in which survival is at stake only the saint or the person comsumed with ambition pursues a subordinating desire. Put this way I realized I had been unable to live the Jesuit life as St. Ignatius, our founder, envisioned it.

Ignatius Loyola lays it out in very simple terms and proposes it as God's plan for every human person. Man, he states, is created to reverence, praise and serve God and by this means to save his soul. All other things are created to help man do this. Hence they are to be used inasmuch as they contribute to this end and dispensed with inasmuch as they hinder this end. Therefore man must make himself indifferent to all things.

Ideally, of course, one writes this plan in the first person and concretizes the goal. I should have been able to say--I am created to be a Jesuit priest

nd all other things are ordered to helping me to be a
esuit priest. I shall follow my desires only insofar
s they help me reach this goal.

It suddenly became clear that the ambitious busi-
essman or artist or scientist may embrace an identical
rdering in his life. I am determined to be a million-
ire--a great sculptor, a great scientist. Everything
lse must be made to help me achieve this goal.

I was discovering again the difference between
eaning and truth. Commitment to any goal with such a
onsuming desire that other desires are subordinated
o it harmonizes a person with intense meaning. The
ind of person one becomes and the measure of genuine
ulfillment and happiness experienced depend, however,
n truth: is one's goal truly humanly fulfilling?

Although I knew I lacked the strength to live un-
er any subordinating desire I felt strongly drawn to
ry to understand how such a life becomes structured.
t might help to understand how the subordinating de-
ire functions. Whether the subordinating desire is
oving service of God or the determination to make mon-
y or be an artist, in all such instances one is, I
ensed, 'seized' by the goal. The desire is so absorb-
ng that the experience is best described as a 'being
eized', rather than a deliberate choice, even though
t must indeed be freely submitted to and embraced.
et it is not that simple.

No love becomes a true love without conflict and
hoice. 'Being seized' by a goal does not mean other
esires cease. Inevitably desires and loves conflict.
 habit of preferring the chosen goal must be estab-
ished. And implicit at least is the intellectual con-
iction that other desires really have their value in
elation to this primary desire. Extraordinary self-
iscipline is required, after considerable sacrifices.
ne cannot reach the freedom which pursuit of one goal
ives without habitually saying 'no' to one's other de-
ires. Loneliness, sacrifice of friendship's delights,
ard, hard work are customarily part of the price. The
armony, the wholeness, the freedom results from a dia-
ectical process: positive growth in love of the goal
and negative control of other desires.

In other words 'being seized' by the goal is not
immediately effective. One has to grow in such love
and in control of conflicting desires precisely to allow the principal love to expand. Initially a period of

51

asceticism is required which should develop into an easy habit of correctly choosing. For the saint God becomes more and more real through prayer. For the artist or entrepreneur concern for the goal comes to control more and more of one's consciousness through various means. The self-denial, penances, mortifications of the saint function negatively to achieve freedom to love God. These are well known and frequently looked upon as folly. Seeking wealth or fame demands as spartan a regime as the saints. We tend to ignore or to take for granted as worthwhile the self-denial, sacrifices, even the great risks entailed by these more tangible goals.

This asceticism nurtures the harmonization of the person by muting other desires. It need not entail a loss of the desire. If my love of X grows in intensity, love of Y may seem to be lessened even though it may not have changed at all. The artist's preference for solitude prompted by love of his art need not exclude love of his friends. As the love of God intensifies, love of one's friends need not change, though it may be muted. Very often the preferential love of a marriage partner is expressed by muting or not allowing to develop love for someone else.

This muting of desires results both from increasing the love of the goal and from non-indulgence under motivation of the primary love. In the latter tactic the initial choices may well be difficult. Habits, however, make difficult things easy and can in time make them desirable. Even what repels can come to be willingly embraced as one's attitude changes. A saintly priest once outlined for me the stages of spiritual progress in the chronically sick. His insights were born from thirty years of crippling tuberculosis. The first step, he explained, is to acknowledge that one is not going to be cured. This many never achieve, he claimed. In the second stage the patient accepts the sickness as God's will. One can finally come to want it, not masochistically of course, but precisely in joining one's will with God's. In an analogous way dislike or difficulty in choices may be overcome in any life and even made desirable.

It was becoming clear just how a subordinating desire harmonizes a person in his desires and structures an intensely meaningful life. Always seeking the one thing one loves, rather than being dissipated in pursuit of many desires, fills life with intense meaning. Competing desires have been muted. But more, the determinant for choice even in these other desires becomes not the intrinsic appeal, but the contribution to

the goal of the subordinating desire. In the case
when the object of choice has no intrinsic appeal, perhaps is even repulsive, it still has appeal because of
its relation to the primary love. In this way the subordinating desire pervades all desires. No wonder the
person experiences harmony and drive.

Monomania, of course, always lurks in the wings of
the life harmonized under a subordinating desire. True,
"man does not live by bread alone", but man does live
by bread. No matter how spiritualized a person becomes,
he remains human and never ceases to function completely as a man without harm to himself or to society.
Similar harm and diminishment can befall the artist,
scientist or seeker of wealth.

Saint, artist, entrepreneur experience intensely
meaningful lives for the same reason: their subordinating desire so pervades all their desires that in
essence they are always seeking that which they most
love. There is the same expansion of that subordinating desire and the muting of other desires. But neither
is the process totally the same nor is the kind of person who results the same. I might mention again that
meaning is not happiness. The fruit of happiness grows
from truth not from meaning. I reached these conclusions from imagining a pure form of each kind of life
under such subordinating desires. It does not matter
that the pure form may never be realized. We all know
people who at least move in the direction of the pure
form and illustrate the benefits and harms attendant
upon such lives.

I had a student in an ethics course who, I sensed,
might well stand for the typically ambitious man. He
had set his material goals high and definite. This
predetermined what he considered worth learning and to
that extent made learning certain subjects impossible.
His only reason for taking my course was to fulfill a
core requirement. I often wondered if he might well
succeed in earning his first million by the age of 35
and suddenly discover he did not know why he wanted it.

If this boy Russ were actually to structure his
life with wealth as his subordinating desire, I could
imagine how it might develop. His initial ambition
would find itself tested by conflict with his desires
to have a good time, to be one of the boys. Only gradually would the pursuit of wealth or of the means to
acquire it come to pervade his life. Once having chosen, for example, to make his way in industry or bank-

ing he would acquire the skills needed. Friends would
be cultivated to help him get ahead. Experiencing the
need of a woman and perceiving that marriage improved
his chances for success he would look not for love but
for financial advantages. Gradually everything he encountered would be ordered to make him wealth. If
choices involved sacrifice of friendship and loyalty,
they would force him to more complete commitment to the
dollar god. As he developed into this one-dimensional
man, economic man, other dimensions of his person would
be unexpressed. Yet on the other hand many desires
might not be so muted as to exclude indulgence. Sexual
indulgence, getting drunk might in the right circumstances not interfere with business, in fact might help.

Russ could live an intensely meaningful life, one
indeed in which he might feel he was very happy. The
pursuit of immediately challenging goals as well as the
overall goal of economic success might suffice even till
death. He must, of course, never question his values.
It is essential that the distorted superficial image of
man successfully dazzle Russ's sense of what it is to be
a man. He must never recognize the emptiness, the inadequacy of such limited, contingent goals. For Russ is
more than economic man. He is social, lover, artist,
part of nature, son of God. I can not believe Russ could
use friends and wife instead of experiencing friendship
and love and yet be truly happy. Unless a person expresses a certain number of the essential dimensions of
his drive-to-be he cannot experience happiness. Tragedy
is built into Russ's life. He has to play the game with
himself that his goal is absolute enough to warrant risk-
ing his entire life. Possibly the suicides of successful men may be laid at the door of sudden revelation that
it has been a game.

I am imagining Russ committed to wealth as a desire
which pervades and subordinates all other desires. This
is very different from the pursuit of wealth as a dominant desire. The same is true for my example of the artist, Ernst.

Art can capture a person's heart as a subordinating
desire and function much the way wealth can. Perhaps
the reason a life with art as the subordinating desire
appears more ennobling than Russ's is that unlike wealth
art intrinsically perfects the person and is in principal ordered to benefit others. It can however fail the
person just as wealth does when it poses as an absolute
and as an adequate fulfillment of the person.

I can imagine Ernst discovering some talent with
words and letting the desire to be a writer expand. The
discipline required might very soon have forced him to
choose definitely to be a writer. As he became fascina-
ted with the tools of his trade he risked substituting
expression for being. When becoming the great novelist
began to organize the meaning of his life subordinating
all other desires, then friendship, love, society came
to be "used" for his art. Instead of loving a woman
Ernst might well have desired the experience of loving
to help him to write. I question whether he then really
could experience love. Along with the risk of substituting expression for being, Ernst is building tragedy
into his life. He is more than artist. Fulfillment of
the human person, happiness involve the expression and
development of at least essential dimensions of his
drive-to-be. Ernst is not only artist, but animal, social being, lover, economic man, son of God. Unless
these dimensions find expression tragedy is eating its
way through Ernst's life. Living for his art, the day
he wakes to recognize his artistic powers have gone all
meaning will flee and perhaps only the gun remain.

I focused upon Walter to illustrate the saint, for
he is the only one I have met who might in my judgment
possibly be a saint. Yet it became palpably evident
that I was no more sure I understood the saint's ordering of life under the subordinating desire of love of
God than I was that I knew what went on in the artist or
entrepreneur. There is no one lifestyle God uses to
lead a person to sanctity. Hence no easy way to point
out the saint or his ways. Not every one who leads a
spiritual life gives evident signs of doing so. Even
the genuinely spiritual need not be wise and in the
truth. And it is necessary for success to be in the
truth. Furthermore, to be a saint does not mean to be
perfect as a man. Hence there are bound to be dimensions of the saint which fail to find expression. Finally, perfect happiness is experienced only in heaven.
I indeed see sanctity as the fulfillment of the person
precisely as a person and hence as the surest way to
happiness. But pursuit of holiness in no way eliminates
the human condition with its chances, its failures, its
sufferings. It does however transform them, bringing
more joy on earth than any other way of life.

Walter exemplified this. He had been a tuberculosis victim for 25 years when I began to cultivate
him. My efforts were deliberate for I had heard he was
very holy. After some months of regular visiting as a
first year seminarian I concluded his reputation was

merely that--a reputation. I surmised people said he
was holy because they thought he ought to be. Just before Christmas and shortly after his sister had died,
Walter was in a mellow mood and the wall came down. I
saw something of the real Walter. Not only did his
faith, his trust, his union with God reveal themselves
but also his humanness. He coped very well with his
sickness but he had never been able to accept with ease
the dependence on others. It really hurt him to sense
people were visiting him not from personal interest but
from some sense of obligation. He loved news and "scut-
tle-butt". He laughed a lot and enjoyed movies.

If Walter ever let desire for God subordinate all
his desires--and I never knew him well enough to say he
did--then I imagine some such growth as this. He was
certainly a typical American boy. He grew up loving
sports and was particularly good at baseball. I presume his faith was established and nurtured in a religious family. Growing out of a prayerful, religious and
moral adolescence came a vocation to become a Jesuit
priest. Although he laid the foundation for vibrant
commitment to God in the noviceship I suspect it was
only through experienced humiliation and suffering that
he recognized God calling him to heroic love. He would
differ from Russ and Ernst in the muting of desires.
For every aspect of life would be important to Walter.
He was trying to become perfect not as artist, not as
economic man, but precisely as man, the beloved creature
of God. Thus all desires would be muted under the subordinating desire to know and serve God. While he sacrificed the experience of marriage and children, and to
that extent was diminished in his humanness, he not only
expanded in love of God and friends but linked such sacrifice with loving response to God's invitation to do so.
I believe Walter grew to accept and desire his sickness
by joining his will with God's. Thus love of God became very concrete as loving acceptance of the life of
a tubercular victim. This was his vocation. It gave
meaning to all he did and all he accepted--all he could
not do. Love of others grew--care grew. Patience, hu-
mility, understanding, wisdom all grew. His was a meaningful life, his was a happy life even in his suffering.

Russ, Ernst and Walter ended up very different
kinds of persons. And only Walter was truly happy. Yet
all three experienced intensely meaningful lives for
all three had one love pervading all they did subordinating all their other desires. I felt I understood
how this subordinating desire so controlled

the constellation of desires as to let each person be consciously one and whole. This is the road to greatness. The risks involved need not lead to tragedy. But few are strong enough to be great, to subordinate all their desires under one harmonizing goal, fewer still are wise enough to be happy in their greatness.

I am not among the great or the wise. I knew the meaning in my life did not come from the control of a subordinating desire. Yet my life was without doubt meaningful. There must be another way of harmonizing desires. As I weighed the things which counted in my life I concluded that my vocation to be a Jesuit priest was the most significant of my desires. I felt I could designate it as my dominant desire. While I had experienced something of "being seized" and I had practiced some of the asceticism required to develop and expand the desire to be Jesuit priest, I definitely had not been driven to achieve like Russ, Ernst or Walter. The key to the difference I found in the muting of desires.

Muted desires even when indulged in are pervaded by the subordinating desire. In this way it can be said that one is always following the central desire. In my case desires were in many cases muted, but many were not and were enjoyed for themselves. The control by the dominant desire was exercised through its function as a negative norm. Any desire could be followed provided it did not jeopardize the dominant desire. Reflective gazing on my life revealed two other aspects of the dominant desire which helped to explain how it harmonizes. It commands most of a person's time and energy. It is what makes the person the kind of person he is. I began to see these three aspects as criteria of a dominant desire. They are not, however, a facile litmus paper device. Rather they serve as pointers, now one, now another being invoked, which allow an intuitive grasp of the distinctiveness of the person.

Studying two friends of mine in the light of these three criteria confirmed my description. Oliver is a doctor, happily married, the father of four children. His dominant desire is to be husband and father. He has always wanted to be a doctor; it might even be questioned whether his dominant desire might not be to be a doctor rather than husband-father. Certainly he functions better as a doctor because marriage completes him as a person. Profession blends without conflict with the desire to be husband-father. But if a serious conflict were ever to force a radical choice between wife and profession, profession would yield to wife. The

opposite is indeed conceivable, but it would not be my
friend Oliver. The man who is husband-father and in as-
dition is a doctor differs markedly from the man who is
doctor and in addition is husband and father. Oliver is
the former.

The order in his life is clear. He loves his wife
Gwendolyn and with her loves their children. The dominant desire to be husband-father leads first to the expression of love of, and the nurturing and deepening of
union with, Gwen and the children. These activities
directly express the desire. But countless other activities take their meaning from relation to this desire.
He devotes considerable time and energy planning what
may please Gwen and help her and the children enjoy
themselves and grow happily as persons. On him lies the
burden of providing for the basic needs of the entire
family. This commands much of his time and attention.
Fortunately society richly rewards his service as a doctor so that provision is no great problem.

Since this is a dominant, not a subordinating desire, numerous other desires are freely indulged in.
Friendships, cards, sports, a certain amount of political involvement find expression to the extent they do
not endanger his desire to be husband-father as concretized in the activities this desire has structured. As
a matter of fact various dimensions of Oliver find expression in these other desires so that he has become
a more complete person. Desires for other women, of
course, are muted for they conflict with his desire for
Gwen. The function of negative norm also operates when
arguments with his partners make him want to break away
until he recognizes the harm that would come to Gwen
and the children.

I sense a genuine harmony in Oliver. He is one
and whole, Gwen's husband and the children's father at
all times. Indeed he is doctor at all times. It is not
that he does the husbandly or fatherly or doctor-thing,
he is husband-father-doctor at all times. Whether he
is dealing with a patient, writing a medical paper, or
drinking at a party, he is husband-father-doctor. Because he is harmonized as one he acts with ease, all
his desires ordered. He "does his thing". He wants to
do what he does.

His dominant desire set Oliver in a definite direction and as habits developed the expression of this desire, he became that kind of person: husband-father-
doctor. But the kind of person, the role is played in

58

individual, distinctive style. For the choices have been free and the grasp of the purpose of the choices intelligent. So he carries himself with ease. If he had chosen the profession or followed the dominant desire for extrinsic motives such as status or to please parents, or if he had locked himself into expected role characteristics without intelligent structuring and sensitive assessment he would not be so liberated.

Speaking more generally, in even the ideal development of a person in the role specified by the dominant desire, there may well be attendant diminishment of the person. Certain dimensions of the drive-to-be, certain desires may not be developed or indulged in. Limited energy or family problems may require, for example, muting desires for music, or art. Furthermore being made one and whole through the harmonization of desires gives one the power to cope with responsibilities, pressures and suffering, but is no guarantee against them.

No man lives alone. The prevailing culture influences the way the dominant desire works itself out in specific activities. Today it is difficult to escape technocratic systematization and the custom of postponing enjoyment. Oliver's children as well as his own and Gwen's sensitivity have awakened him to the need to insure that present enjoyment of what he is doing function as one index of choices.

Oliver has so much going for him because his profession blends in so well with his dominant desire and is handomely rewarded by society. He is so well harmonized because he genuinely desires the work which provides for the basic needs of the family. Many, however, find meaning in part of their lives structured under their dominant desire, but have to provide for their basic needs by work they dislike. My friend Vincent typifies so many. Like Oliver he finds rich meaning and satisfaction in being husband and father. He loves his wife, Alice, and devotes his life to her and their four children, providing for their needs, their happiness, their growth, preparing them for life. Being with his family, enjoying them, planning for the future of all and each is what he wants out of life.

To that extent Vincent's life is structured under the same dominant desire as Oliver's. The way each provides for the basic needs creates a marked difference. Oliver so enjoys being a doctor that he feels he is a doctor first to serve people and if in the process he makes a living that is great. Vincent finds no intrinsic appeal in his work. The only reason he works for

General Motors is that it pays enough to provide for the basic needs and other desires of his family. Only profit provides motivation to put up with the dullness and repulsiveness of the work. A large segment of his life is not harmonized. In a sense he is two persons. One has meaning, the other endures.

Vincent has come to grips with this. By changing his own attitude, by accepting the uncongenial aspects of the work situation and focusing on companionship and money benefits, by religious reinterpretation and acceptance he has found a way to live with it. The fact that so many have to learn to live with such unsatisfactory conditions warrants radical rethinking of our economic system. But my concern remains with Vincent: he certainly enjoys a meaningful life. Who can measure a person's interior drive and happiness? Yet so far as I can penetrate he simply is unable to harmonize his life as fully as Oliver: a large part is bracketed.

Nonetheless both Vincent and Oliver illustrate the life made meaningful under a dominant desire. The insight I had caught pondering over harmonization of desires in general rang true in itself. But testing it on the lives of two of my friends helped me to understand it better and to be confirmed in its truth.

For both the dominant desire to be husband-father blended all their desires in harmony. This desire expressed itself by commanding most of their time and energy. It differed, however, from the control of a subordinating desire. This latter mutes all desires at least as regards choice and thus pervades all desires. Being husband-father allowed other desires to flourish unless they conflicted with this dominant desire. Thus instead of pervading all desires it functioned as a negative norm. Finally being husband-father determined the kind of person each became, in an individualized way of course.

I felt I understood this second constitutive element in the meaningful life. I could write that summary now with conviction. I can act only if I am. I can be only if I am one. I can act with meaning and desire only if I am meaningful to myself. I can be meaningful to myself only if I am consciously one. I can be consciously one only if in my desires I am harmonized as one under either a subordinating or dominant desire.

I had come to feel secure in my grasp of the two essential constitutive elements in a meaningful life:

an overarching meaning and the harmonization of desires.
Long hours of reflective gazing had been spent before
they and their functioning stood sharply revealed. Almost in the process of uncovering the other elements,
however, I recognized both their importance and function.
The need to provide for the expression of a sufficient
number of the dimensions of a person, the contribution
of responsible freedom and the reason for a wise selection of activities expressive of all these are easily
understood. Likewise no extended thought was needed to
grasp the importance of living within habits and institutions yet remaining sensitive to any shackling effects.
I have already illustrated the importance of the way one
provides for basic needs in view of how this blends into
the whole of one's life. It seemed to me no further explanation was needed. Anyone concerned about meaning in
his life would, of course, do well to scrutinize each of
these elements within his own life. As for myself I felt
ready to test my analysis: if it could explain just why
pain made my life non-meaningful, I would feel it was
confirmed. As I moved in that direction it became clear
I would first have to crystalize for myself just how the
elements blended and structured meaning into my life.
What is it to be a Jesuit? Somehow I sensed the answer
would be important in the final explanation which my
analysis would bring to the effects of pain.

CHAPTER FIVE

Autobiography of a Dominant Desire-I

Nothing exciting had stirred me in my discovery of the harmonization of desires. This surprised me for the discovery that the Blessed Trinity needed me to 'experience' my unique responses and contributions to life had so fired me that I was inclined to remain satisfied with just the overarching meaning. Perhaps the difference lay in the fact that I had come to grips with the actual overarching meaning which made sense of the desires I experienced but casual recognition that my dominant desire was to be a Jesuit priest had allowed me to remain detached in my analysis of how a dominant desire functions to harmonize one's life. Now I found I had to reopen the question. Just how are my desires harmonized? Do I actually desire to be a Jesuit priest? What does it mean? Unless this became real to me I knew I might well have uncovered the constitutive elements of a meaningful life but I would be unable to apply the insights to explain the loss of meaning in my life.

Everything became more personal and I felt drawn to let my life pass in review before me. How did I arrive at the harmony in my life? In grammar school, I can recall, I told a nun that I wanted to be a priest. When the original seed had been planted I don't know. But certainly the faith and religious atmosphere of my family, my close relatives, friends and the nuns and priests whom I knew well and respected definitely nurtured the desire to be a priest--although I do not remember much talk about it or encouragement, much less any urging. It strikes me as strange that young people feel called to be priests or doctors or scientists without any real understanding of what it means to be a priest or doctor or scientist.

The desire to be a priest grew during the exciting, maturing years of high school. One of the nuns became a close friend and encouraged me to grow in prayer. Father John McGlinchey, one of my teachers, had significant influence on me. Poverty kept me from any sort of sheltered life. From the fifth grade through my first year in college I caddied. Exposed though I was to conflicting religious views and significantly different moral values and practices, somehow I never felt any real challenge on these matters. Perhaps an internalized ghetto can operate when the exterior ghetto is breached. The loves I experienced never really called into question what God wanted me to do. Prayers, penances and reflection increased as the need to decide pressed to a point. In my freshman year at Boston College I made the decision to enter the Jesuits. I did not have any clear idea of the difference between a religious and a diocesan priest. Nor would it have mattered much to me at the time if the Jesuits had refused me. I would have applied to the diocesan seminary. It was during the noviceship that I actually received my vocation to embrace the religious life as a priest.

How different it is actually to experience the events of one's life and to recollect these same events after 30 odd years of lived through experiences with their effects known. In the summer of 1936 I arrived at Shadowbrook, the novitiate in Lenox, Mass. Not quite twenty I had the vibrant emotion of commitment to God and the shyness and insecurity of a young man totally ignorant of the life he was entering upon. In memory's eye the opening months blended intense religious consolation, deep aloneness, and physical fatigue. Early rising, disciplined work, but perhaps especially tense determination to do everything perfectly erased fifteen or twenty pounds from my chubby body. It took me eight years to regain normal weight. I was away from home for the first time and among total strangers. While the structures, the sureness of those in charge and the manifest concern and efforts of all to be friendly provided an atmosphere of security, years of growth, of personal friendships, of experienced satisfaction passed before loneliness was replaced with a general feeling of being at home. At the same time, however, rich consolation flooded my soul, bringing joy and assurance I was on the road God wanted.

As I rolled back the years in an effort to recapture my responses to the noviceship experiences I was penetrated with a sense of awe. What I had uncovered so far was relatively simple. From within the lived experience of a life successfully structured with meaning I had intuited the constitutive elements which gave that meaning. I now ambitioned insight into the process of structuring meaning into a life. Becoming is far more mysterious than being.

My life has never been so meaningful as it now is. In fact I sense it is opening into a new level of meaning, just as my present level is distinct from that of a few years ago. Each of these levels, however, involve

the experience of my life being meaningful. I can uncover different levels, but I reach a first, not easily
pinpointed, when I actually had succeeded in structuring
a meaningful life. Previous to this level my life was
meaningful in hope, in the process of trying to become
meaningful.

I think I reached the level of being whole, being
Jesuit-priest-professor, about 1960-65. All the years
before this I was in the process of becoming this Jesuit-
priest-professor. I really had not become whole previous
to this. About this time I was secure in who I was, I
found that my different roles blended and were satisfying. Activities, habits, friendships had been established. Change remained the law and with change there
is always risk. Sometimes growth, sometimes regression.
But in general it was a question of going to another
level of being meaningful, not of becoming meaningful.
There is in principle, I believe, no limit to growth
until one is perfectly united with God in the beatific
vision. Such openness to growth should, I hope, keep my
life vibrant and eager.

Before that vague date between 1960 and 1965 the
meaning in my life was meaning in the immediate appealing, based on youthful openness, energy and hope that
what I was doing would result in a meaningful life. I
ambitioned being a Jesuit-priest. I did not know whether being a Jesuit priest would prove to be meaningful or
not. The process of striving to become that kind of
person was meaningful precisely as the process of becoming. At some point the becoming had succeeded and
I could say (though I never did) I now am Jesuit priest
and it is good.

The young man or woman who desires to be a doctor
must go through a similar process. The years of inten-
sive study and training may be meaningful, either appealing in themselves or at least accepted as necessary
to the goal, precisely as the process of becoming a doctor. But the risk remains--becoming is not being. He
or she does not know whether being doctor will prove
meaningful or not. At some point he will complete the
process and experience that he is doctor and find it
meaningful to be a doctor or not.

I sensed how important it was that I try to capture
the process by which my desires became harmonized. I
thought of the young people I knew and realized they
simply could not see the question of meaning as I did.
I was trying to understand the state of being meaningful

looking from within a life successfully structured as meaningful. They had to focus upon the process of becoming, of structuring lives which would be meaningful. Becoming is not being. Becoming can be understood in the light of being. Being cannot be understood in the light of becoming. Possibly my experiences might provide some helpful suggestions if I could recapture what happened to me in the process of becoming Jesuit-priest

Far from being enthusiastic about what help I migh give the young I soberly realized how little control I had going through the process. I had been confused, un sure, so very lucky and blessed in what happened and what did not happen. Everyone must grow from within, everyone has to risk. Still what happened to me might provide some hints.

Most young people in their upper teens experience anguish as they search to discover what they should do with their lives. Two concerns face them: what to become, how to provide for basic needs. A young man, for instance, may assume he wants to be husband and father and focus upon choosing a career to provide for basic needs. Until he commits himself to a particular woman he has hardly begun to structure meaning into his life. Still he probably pursues activities which appeal or excite and which may or may not be building toward anything. Time allows the sifting of possibilities until the way of providing for basic needs which appeals or which he realizes is the best available looms decisively.

Such broad strokes suffice to portray the early period of the normal process of developing. But the young today face a more acute problem. The accepted life-styles for the husband-father role as well as for providing for basic needs are under challenge and in many instances do not appeal. In fact many seem to make living with expanded consciousness or at least with the experience of as much delight as possible their dominant or even subordinating desire. Drugs and leisure become ordered to this. People are experimenting with various forms of communal living.

In recent years the affluence of our society has permitted a prolonged period of maturing without positive relating to the established forms of providing for necessities. At some time, however, the young must take a stand: opt into the establishment, work against it, go in far enough to provide for one's needs but structure one's life-style independently, or live para-

sitically upon it. The way one provides for basic needs
is so important and must blend harmoniously with one's
dominant desire that the difficulty the young now face
is evident. Hence not only the anguish, but also the
ventures into new life-style, some obviously harmful,
some with definite promise.

Underlying these challenges to traditional life-
styles vibrates a rejection, or at least a distrust, of
traditionally held values and truths. Rooting this rejection itself pulses a change in consciousness, a change
in the very way to assess truths and values. Not even
those young who favor the traditional forms escape these
subtle changes. No one is unaffected.

Our young have to find answers for the same questions as we did--what to become, how to provide for
basic needs--but without the security people of my generation enjoyed. It was my third year in high school, I
believe, when I sensed I should be reaching a decision.
Did I really have a vocation to be a priest? How could
I know? I prayed more, I discussed it a little bit.
This very effort kept my life meaningful at its core. I
enjoyed most things I got involved in; my studies were
meaningful. Why the former made life meaningful is
understandable; the latter however, was the result of
trust. In my trust there was no question but that the
studies were wisely planned for my future. No need of
investigating, planning. Just work at what was assigned.
Such trust provided peace and contentment during the
time I gradually reached the decision to apply to the
Jesuits and to begin the positive process of structuring
my life as Jesuit-priest.

Contrast my experience with that of a young friend
of mine. A fun loving, athletically gifted young man he
spent his freshman year at college in soul searching.
He reached, in the secrecy of his own counsel, the decision to chart his program in such a way that if he decided to be a doctor he would have the prerequisites.
If he decided, on the other hand, not to be a doctor, he
would have a major in another field. He revealed his
ambitions to no one. Perhaps he refused to risk laughter in case his marks made his ambitions ridiculous. On
his own he had to work out the selection of courses
suitable for this difficult program.

For three years he lived out of character, isolat-
ing himself, passing up fun, slaving at the books. Was
his life meaningful? I would guess it was more intensely meaningful than the few years preparatory to my opt-

ing positively into the process which structured meaning into my life. His exercise of freedom and his responsibility intensified meaning. But the very need of
responsibly managing his own life, of living out of character, I would assume, provided less peace, less joy
than I possessed. In any event his secret hopes were
realised and after graduation he was accepted into a
distinguished medical school.

He is finding the process of becoming a doctor
meaningful. He cannot know whether being a doctor will
measure up to his expectations. While he knows he wants
to be husband-father and, I feel sure, wants this as his
dominant desire, he has not yet met the girl whom he
would want as wife and mother of his children. It is
young people like him whom I hope to help a little by
crystalizing my experience of structuring meaning into
my life.

As I compared myself with this young friend two
important differences impressed me. His dominant desire,
I have said, is to be husband-father. Until he discov-
ers the right girl he will be unable to shape his life.
And how does he know she is the right girl or whether
chance errors or emotional hurts will harm or prevent
union? Even granted the right choice, will they grow
together? Will she truly desire to be wife and mother
as he develops being husband-father? While the religious has no more assurance than my friend that he will
grow within his permanent commitment he does have two
years of noviceship to try out the life before committing himself in vows. Courtship and guidance must substitute in the case of marriage.

Secondly the process of incorporation during the
noviceship as well as the years of growth into the community took place in a very different atmosphere than
my friend is experiencing in medical school. He is
not at all sure he wants to be molded into the kind of
person the medical school envisions. Without trust he
goes his own way selectively following directives. I
entered into these formative experiences with complete
docility based upon utter trust.

I do not find it easy to discern the stages of my
becoming Jesuit-priest. But I think there were three.
The first, and most critical, was the incorporation into the Society of Jesus culminating in the profession
of vows two years after I entered. Many years of
growth followed, years of intense study under strict
supervision interspersed with regency, a time of prac-

tical experience in the Society's work, teaching in my case, but also years of establishing human ties as well as of growing familiarity with Jesuit life. Ordination to the priesthood climaxed this second stage. Growing continued through tertianship, graduate studies, teaching assignment until that indiscernible point when I could say I am Jesuit-priest.

Trying to recapture what happened to me in that critical process of incorporation I recalled what a young wife and mother once told me. She revealed that her greatest concern in the early part of their marriage was how Jim would react to the illumination that she was only an ordinary person. When the light did dawn they had so grown together that it did not matter. I can only imagine that the process of becoming a two-in-one person of marriage must involve a radical upheaval of perspectives and values and a restructuring of conscious responses similar to what I experienced. In both cases strong emotional satisfaction eases the upheaval. I believe years of growing in respect, in trust, sharing, pain. and joy are experienced before a couple can say--we are one; or the man can say--I am husband-father to this woman and these children. My years of growth until I could say I am Jesuit-priest parallel that experience.

August 14, 1936 brought me to Shadowbrook, a truly beautiful spot overlooking the Stockbridge bowl so I could formally begin my noviceship the next day on the feast of Mary's Assumption. A two-week period, called postulancy (under the fiction of candidates requesting admission), provided an easy introduction to the routine, the customs, the method of prayer, both private and common. It also allowed a sense of camaraderie to begin and generated an increasing desire to belong to the novice community which we watched but did not join.

Receiving the habit marked our entrance into the noviceship. I was introduced gradually to a series of practices whose purpose was to refine my awareness of God's presence and to sensitize my consciousness of being directed by the Holy Spirit. Different forms of prayer, meditation, contemplation, vocal prayers, examination of conscience, the habit of recollection were proposed in instructions and established by practice. Conferences explained the spiritual life, asceticism, the religious life, specifically the Jesuit life. Regular spiritual reading deepened my understanding of all this and provided motivation to desire such a life. A sense of community was being established, persons coming to be liked, loved, esteemed. And belonging to the Jesuits became a matter of pride.

From my present vantage point I recognize a two-fold development in this process of incorporation. The vertical relationship with God who was inviting me to belong to this community was and remains the most important element. In principle every Jesuit belongs to the Society because he is convinced God wants him here. But the horizontal relationship of human ties grows as well.

These two relationships blend together, a pervasive union growing out of the same vision shared, the same interpretation of life embraced, the same goal pursued. The Jesuits are a community of intelligent men freely embracing the same specific way of life. The most influential experience in this process of incorporation into the Society is the thirty days devoted to the Spiritual Exercises of St. Ignatius, the founder of the Society of Jesus. Not only is it an intense praying experience, but it provides the situation for each Jesuit to undergo the fundamental religious experience through which God had shaped St. Ignatius. Jesuits all over the world are united through the shared vision of God's intentions for mankind grasped through the experience of the Spiritual Exercises as interpreted through the Constitutions of the Society in the lived tradition of the community.

October with its autumnal splendor and starlit skies ushered in this "long retreat," thirty days, interrupted three times with a day of quiet relaxation and talking. In complete silence we devoted four hours daily to prayerful penetration of the meaning of life in an orchestrated series of experiences which lead step by step to total, joyful commitment to Jesus Christ The opening days lay out in simple but stark language God's plan of creation and salvation. The logic, presupposing belief in God, the Creator, is inexorable and I was penetrated intellectually and emotionally with the realization of my dependence on God, the consequent need to discover His will for me and with an utter conviction that reasonable living demanded genuine control of all attachments, choosing always what would be most conducive for achieving my goal. Hardly had these convictions seeped into my soul than the reality and horror of sin and sinfulness exploded within me. Remorse flooded my soul and I sobbed in repentance. Joy poured through my entire being after a general confession, for not only did I experience forgiveness but the incredible

love of the God who died for my sins and who had stead-
ily pursued this prodigal son.

About twelve days had accomplished this conviction
and purgation. A "break-day" released nerves and refreshed minds. We returned to the silence to contem-
plate Christ the King inviting us to total service in
His campaign. I thrilled to the call and struggled at
least to want to signalize myself in absolute commitment, whatever that might entail. Contemplating Jesus
in His incarnation, birth, infancy and finding in the
temple I grew to know Him better, to feel more love and
more at ease with Him. This lulled me a bit on the
challenge of commitment. But I was not allowed to elude
the deepened awareness of what it involved. Certain
exercises simply forced me to face up to the challenge.
I felt seared with the searching light of God's looking
at me: do you want to follow my Son in poverty, chastity and obedience? Half-way measures won't do, rationalization won't do. More aware of what the call involved, its cost, I felt not emotionally enthusiastic,
but rather grimly determined to give myself to Christ's
service. Further prayer on Christ in his public life
reassured me. And we had reached the second "break day."

We relaxed, but soberly, aware of how deeply involved we had become. Silence enshrouded us at the end
of the day and we faced the passion and death of Christ.
His suffering and his love pierced into me. My grim
determination to serve Christ dropped the grimness and
became grateful, loving commitment. It was a difficult
section of the retreat and the third "break day" was
welcome.

Meditation on the resurrection and the joy of the
Lord lifted my spirit and I was more sure than ever I
wanted to belong to Christ. The final days were devoted to tasting the love of God experienced in all He
is and does. I felt bathed in love, ready to serve,
confident it would be a joyful way to offer my life.
Looking back thirty-five or more years later I recognize this experience of the Spiritual Exercises as the
most shaping experience in my life. It has affected
my responses to every significant event in my life. Yet
I see its creative force was still seeking form and
could easily have been dissipated if the appropriate
life-style had not been established. Many have made
the Exercises without developing a spiritual life, still
more without becoming Jesuits.

The retreat had broken me open and the seeds of a

new life had been planted. This new life was first of
all an interior life, a sensitized consciousness of what
went on within me: my motives, my emotional and willed
responses, my perspectives. Not every interior life is
a spiritual life. Not every life of faith is an interior life. But when a person lives his faith interiorly
he is living the spiritual life. The spiritual life
may be said to begin when one begins to be led by the
Spirit. As one grows in awareness of the reality of God,
the Blessed Trinity living in a very special union
through the baptized human person, he seeks to understand
life and reality, to shape his values, to make his decisions according to the direction of the Blessed Trinity.
As this direction is usually attributed to the third
Person, he is said to be led by the Holy Spirit. Prayer
to nurture and develop awareness of God's presentce is
obviously a necessity. But it is equally necessary in
order to permeate one's mind with revealed truth, to
'put on the mind of Jesus Christ'. Our Lord's life provides a model for judging the response the Blessed Trinity desires to take through each person in every situation. Ascetical practices liberate the person from in-
stinctual or acquired responses freeing him to follow
God's inspirations.

Clearly the spiritual life is the significantly
Christian life. God leads his people in a thousand ways.
What is common to all is the life of faith. But not many
seem drawn to this interiorized spiritual life. While
God may lead men to the spiritual life in many ways, under his providence men have through the centuries developed a specialized structure for the spiritual life
called the religious life. Though its forms vary, simply and in general the religious life has meant a group
of men or a group of women living together with vows of
poverty, chastity and obedience, under rules to guide
the living out of such vows and in some specific form
of apostolic service. The Church after detailed scru-
tiny gives her approval to the partiular forms of religious life.

The creative force unleashed by my long retreat was
carefuly canalized into an interior, spiritual, Jesuit
life. Our Master of Novices was keenly conscious that
the most exalted, moving experiences require solid convictions as well as basic asceticism to have lasting
effect. Shortly after the retreat he began daily conferences. These dealt in depth with the basic truths
involved in the Exercises, the religious life in general, the constitutions of the Society of Jesus in particular, and the principal practices of the ascetical
life: prayer, penance, recollection and spiritual read-

ing. Thus the serious, intellectual underpinning for
the entire enterprise was provided. But by no means
did he assume that understanding through instruction
would suffice. Guiding him, of course, were the tradi-
tions of Church and Society. Regular periods of meditation were provided. In my case, at least, these normally were discursive, heavily intellectual. I sought
really to understand the truths or to penetrate the mind
and heart of Christ portrayed in the Gospels. Affective
prayer, however, together with devout attendance at Mass,
visits to the Blessed Sacrament, and the rosary provided
truly religious experience. Thus the process did not
remain merely intellectual but nurtured a response of
the total person. The cultivation of silence, recollection, which proved taxing, and of penances, both prescribed and voluntary, made one face the reality of what
he was believing and created a silencing of the soul conducive to the encounter with God in formal periods of
prayer or whenever God might break in.

Examination of conscience, twice a day, and regular
personal interviews with the Master of Novices served to
sensitize my conscience, check progress, individualize
direction and keep me earnest about acquiring the habits
proper to this religious way of living. For we were
living as though we had made the vows of poverty, chastity and obedience.

I think I can say that for the next few years I
lived with intense meaning, my desires harmonized under
a subordinating desire. Truly and totally believing God
had created and called me to be a Jesuit I gave myself
to the life. There is a profound psychological strategy in religious vows. Youngster that I was it was not
a question of understanding but of giving myself to this
strategy. It just worked.

The normal secular life finds itself structured by
conjugal and parental desires, by the desire to acquire
wealth, by the desire to plan one's own life, follow
one's own will. Most of a person's time and energy are
consumed in such desires. The vows of chastity, poverty, and obedience block these channels of the drive-to-
be and force one to turn and face God. When these powerful drives for marriage, wealth and independence are
muted, the desire replacing them must be extremely important. In this way the religious life creates the
situation to center one's energies upon the spiritual
life.

As in most human strategies this goal can be thwar-

73

ted by compromise and rationalization. It proved effective for me, however, in the noviceship and for a few
more years. Marriage was not even considered, concern
for money, a job, preparation for a job never entered
my mind. Docile to direction I wanted only to do God's
will. This desire to do God's will became a driving
force, subordinating all other desires. I undertook
extra penances, I followed rules and directives fierce-
ly--for they were God's will. I threw myself into every
task assigned. Recreations were additional areas of
seeking God's will. Personal relations were guided by
signs of God's will. More than once I hurt my mother
and family by gauche, harsh words and actions, all
prompted by good intentions.

By personal experience I have learned not to identify a meaningful with a fulfilled, happy life. I was
turned outside in by these experiences. "Unless the
seed die..." I had to die to the me who had walked
through the front door at Shadowbrook. That "pious
boy" moving under religious sentiment yielded to the
man choosing to do what he discerned as God's will--
in all things; when to pray, what to do, whom to associate with. Spontaneity ceased as I challenged my motives and rooted out self indulgence. Birth in this
context proceeds through dying. Dying is painful.
This was a lonely life for the conscious efforts to
grow made me too artifical to love. Besides, friendship follows the same laws everywhere, no matter how
highly motivated people are, and one of them is the need
of time for friendship to develop.

This may sound strange, but I did not feel unhappy.
In a certain sense I really was happy. But it was the
happiness of intense meaning, of wanting to do what I
was doing, and especially the happiness God's presence
brings. It was, moreover, the happiness of becoming,
not of being. Too many dimensions of my person were
not finding expression to be fully happy. The new me
was in process of being born. It would be years and
after many modifications before I would be whole and
truly happy.

The incorporation into the Society essentially involved this interior transformation but the horizontal
relations were very important. I was with a great
group of people. We laughed a lot and had lots of fun
together. The isolation, geographical and otherwise,
made us very dependent upon one another. Gradually
the new lifestyle I was attempting became more mine
and I was able to be somewhat more spontaneous. In the

summer between my first and second year noviceship I had my mother for a week. Not only was it a precious time for us, we had never looked on one another as two persons like this, but the kindness of superiors helped me to appreciate belonging to the Society. This week became even more precious in recollection for my mother died the following December. I was driven to Boston December 3 and stayed at a Jesuit parish. The way the older Jesuits stationed there accepted me as another Jesuit, their respect, their hospitable attention and concern did as much to make me love the Society as the entire two years at Shadowbrook.

As time went on I grew to look to the Society for everything. Everything was provided by the Society, food, lodging, clothes, medical attention, education. Anything needed the Society provided. From her I took my ideals, my history (the Society began in 1540), my grounds for pride in achievement or for disappointment in failures, my concrete objectives and directions for my formation.

I was ready to pronounce my vows as the two years drew to a close. I had read and studied in my determination to understand the meaning and implication of what I was to solemnly promise. I certainly wanted to belong to this group of men I had joined: the ideal Society with its vision and dedication but also these young men I had been living with.

On August 15, 1938 just before Holy Communion I knelt at the altar in front of the Eucharistic Lord and pronounced my vows of poverty, chastity and obedience and became formally a member of the Society of Jesus. I had reached the first stage in my becoming Jesuit-priest. I was now a Jesuit. But it was more a promise to be a Jesuit than truly being one.

This has not been a pious or preaching excursus but a serious effort to probe the structuring of meaning into my life. Countless religious could testify that they experienced much the same. Those who have not experienced it but to whom Christ is real will be able to understand what happened to me. Unbelievers can ignore the claim of objective truth in my interpretation of my experience. So long as they credit me with sincerity in my beliefs and honest reporting of my experiences they can recognize how meaning came to be structured into my life under a subordinating desire. What will loom as especially important later will be the material activities which make up the life of a religious. The significant ones relate directly or indirectly to God.

CHAPTER SIX

Autobiography of a Dominant Desire-II

My musings and recollections had made the noviceship experience very real once again to me. There was,
however, no nostalgia. Nor did I feel any real regret
as I recalled that such sustained fervor was never to
be repeated, that the desire to do God's will as a
Jesuit was to fade in its power to harmonize all my
other desires from functioning as a subordinating desire to operate rather as a dominant desire. I knew I
was not of heroic cast, one who could live under a subordinating desire. Besides, the intensity and fervor
had developed in an unreal situation. It was not within the real world nor with full awareness of the values
and costs involved that my choices and promises had been
made. But then do we ever truly know what a pledge may
demand when it falls due? The husband or wife with a
crippled partner, did he or she know the marriage vow
would involve this sacrifice? Yet without open-ended
commitment and loyalty love is impossible.

While I did not recognize the fading of the noviceship fervor with nostalgia, neither did I disparage it.
I doubt it was much different than the intense devotion
and promises of early marriage. Both are, I sense, essential stages in the process of love and development.
Unless one is thrown off balance I am not sure he or she
can be opened up to the new way of life. No, I do not
criticize my noviceship but I do judge the years of
growth were not as humanly, as wisely chartered as they
could have been.

The second stage of the process of my becoming
Jesuit priest spanned eleven years, from Juniorate to
ordination. The Juniorate allowed us to start our col-
legiate education, the liberal arts program, within a
structure designed to nurture the spiritual life just
begun but with lessened pressure. Three years of philosophy and sciences followed at Weston. I taught first
year high school for two years of my regency at Fair-
field and obtained a Master's degree in philosophy at
Fordham during my third year. Weston was the scene once
again for my three years of theology and my ordination
to the priesthood.

I grew as a human person in may ways during this

stage. Intellectually I expanded especially in philosophy and theology. My understanding of the spiritual life developed from readings over the years, retreats and experience. But I also learned to eat lobster, drink scotch and smoke. Which may be taken as indicative of how I came to live under a dominant rather than subordinating desire. As freedom increased perseverance at prayer diminished and self-indulgence became more marked. Looking back at the process I think I can say that I had become pretty good as a student, pretty good as a teacher, pretty good as a person, pretty good as a religious. Nothing terrible, nothing great, just mediocre. As appreciation of human pleasures increased I reached the point of wondering whether I should return to theology to become a priest or leave the Society. Although I had no particular woman in heart I saw marriage as beautiful and asked myself the hard question: marriage or priesthood? The question upset me. I reflected, prayed, discussed with a Jesuit priest and came to reaffirm my conviction that God had indeed called me to be a priest.

That the question of marriage arose ten years after I presented myself at Shadowbrook reveals how the desire to do God's will in being a Jesuit priest certainly had ceased to be a subordinating desire. Obviously even its role of harmonizing my life as dominant desire was shaken. Two factors were involved. Sexual and emotional needs are so deep and powerful it is not surprising that these desires remain always something the religious must come to grips with. As a matter of fact seven years later, four years after ordination as a priest, I found myself face to face with the indentical choice. I took final vows as a Jesuit in 1953. Rumors suggested the Church might change its demands for celibacy in her priests. I seriously weighed the idea of leaving the Society. If I were to leave, become a diocesan priest, there was the possibility I might some day be free to marry. If I pronounced final vows that would be impossible, for change in requirements of celibacy would never affect religious priests. My decision to reaffirm my choice of being Jesuit priest in both instances was obviously made with eyes far more open to what I was sacrificing. The second factor was neglect of prayer and a general spiritual mediocrity. The strategy of the vows, as I explained, is to block the channel of these basic desires and thus to force one to focus upon God. Without prayer to keep God real and nurture faith and service how could the channel remain blocked?

The more I reflected on this matter the more I
placed the blame on myself, on my failure to meet the
challenge of continual growth through discerning choices
between natural inclinations and the demands of my commitment in faith to this religious life. I wonder, however, if I would have met the challenge better had three
changes been made in my formation. I wish I had been
alerted to the fact of growth in prayer in the direction of contemplation and been trained to emphasize contemplation in action rather than formal periods of
prayer. Focus upon growth and upon the effort to live
a life of faith can make one keenly aware of the need
of the formal periods of prayer. Such experience of
need gives meaning to them and can motivate perserver-
ance in them.

Secondly, greater freedom might have been provided
for and encouraged which would have developed the sense
of responsible direction of my own life. The fact is
that superiors planned practically every step of our
program. The tremendous motivation stirred up in the
noviceship was poured into precise molds. These molds
were well selected, the 'best' available programs and
sources to develop us as perfectly as possible. Risk
of failure was to be kept at a minimum. Avoiding such
risk they risked the development of creative freedom.
In my case at least they lost. While I worked hard at
every task I approached everything as 'the next thing'
to be done without the drive that free choice and desire imparts. Freedom is the condition needed for re-
leasing the drive-to-be. Without freedom no initiative.
Without initiative no greatness. Although freedom and
release of the drive-to-be of a non-gifted man will
never produce greatness, still without freedom mediocrity is assured.

Apart from the regency period my life in the years
of formation were too artificial. Like an engine idling
I never seemed to be doing anything. I was always preparing. Passing over that problem I come to the third
and most serious change I wish had been made in my formation. It has to do with the understanding of the relation of the religious life to the entire human enterprise. Only recently have I come to relate my life to
the goals of the family of man. This has made my life
more real, more human.

At issue is the understanding of the function of
religion itself in human development, the relation of
Christ and his Church to earlier religions and finally
the role of the religious life in the Church. I came

to see that the Jesuits are not important. The family
of man is important. The Church of Christ is important.
Whatever value the Jesuits may have must come from their
contribution to the work of the Church for the family of
man.

If Mead is right man did not become a 'self' until
society and language simultaneously emerged. Only with
'selves' did the problem of meaning become important.
The survival of the self and of society required meaning for the frightful experiences of death, of suffering, of chance, indeed for the total experience of life
itself. Religious feelings of encounter with the in-
visible and the transcendent articulated in myth provided such meaning. Assuming God's initiative, something like this, I submit, lies at the root of religion.

Judaism was a unique religion with the distinctive
elements of faith, of a conviction in God's historical
intervention, of future rather than past orientation.
Jesus Christ is pivotal in the history of religion, for
the Judaic religion was purified, transfused, fulfilled
by Jesus, and in this form spread through the world.
Contrary to the outre interpretations of Bonhoeffer's
writings, Christianity is the purification and perfection of religion.

Man, then, in his struggles to develop this universe and humanize it is not alone nor has he assumed
this task on his own. He received it as an assignment
from God to be co-creator of the universe. The creative love of the Blessed Trinity embraces primarily
the entire family of man. Making the Jewish nation
(or later, the Christian community) a chosen race
(community) was God's way of loving and benefiting all
men. By becoming man God inserted Himself more completely into history, bringing a new life, a new power, a
new freedom into the world. This new life empowers man
to accomplish the humanizing of the universe, so trans-
forming man that his task is rather to christmanize
the universe. Man can only be fulfilled in and through
this new life brought by Christ. The Church, then, is
ordered to the family of man, to bestow and nurture this
new life.

Out of such a perspective grows a stimulating under
standing of the religious life. I am shoulder to shoulder with man in his efforts to develop this universe by
science, technology, industry and the socio-economic,
political structures most suitable for man's happiness
and growth. Knowing man can not accomplish this without

Christ, I try to assist the Church to bring his life
to men. This I do in a distinctive way, together with
all religious, by witnessing by my life to the reality
of Jesus Christ and eternal life. The witnessing rea-
ssures believers and challenges unbelievers. So real
is Jesus Christ that these men and women find joy, freedom and fulfillment in loving Him to the point of sacrificing the normal means and satisfaction most men require. The religious in the ideal is a challenging
enigma: how can anyone be fulfilled as a human person
without marriage, money and independence? Christian
doctrine may strike some as bizarre and incredible.
Success as human persons without normal human means
puzzles and stands as evidence there may be something
to this Christian story. By living my vows and growing
as a human person I am thus contributing much to the
family of man.

Besides this role of witness that all religious
have each community structures its living witness in a
proper form of the Church's service of man. As their
witness assures believers and challenges unbelievers so
their service is for both. Active orders, such as the
Jesuits, become instruments of the Pope and bishops,
communicating and nurturing the life of Christ, preaching and teaching Christ's message. Not infrequently
they play the prophetic role of challenge to existing
structures both in, and distinct from, the Church that
they be truly Christmanizing.

If my life had been viewed as intermeshed in this
way with the human concerns of the family of man, perhaps it would have seemed more important to keep growing. There had, of course, been some growth. Just the
years of living, especially in the academic programs,
expanded me intellectually, culturally and socially.
Regency, through responsibility as a teacher and through
the liberating thought of Dr. Pollock at Fordham, who
made me much more aware of membership in the family of
man, developed me on all dimensions as a fuller human
person. I had definitely grown in love of, and loyalty
to, the Society. And I moved with increasing ease as
a Jesuit. Yet I believe life would have been more stimulating and growth greater had my relationship with the
family of man been underscored.

The retreat before ordination in my third year of
theology made me keenly conscious of the mediocrity per-
meating my life. The retreat director probed a sensitive area with the refrain, "What have you done with the
years? The Society has given you these thirteen years

81

to prepare to be a priest. What have you done with the years?" In the humiliation of realizing my answer to that question it took courage and confidence in God's grace to accept ordination. Only strong, awed conviction that God truly wanted me to be His priest prompted me to go through with it.

Ordination marked a new plateau. It climaxed the second stage of my becoming a Jesuit-priest and launched the final stage until that point when it would have been correct to say "I am Jesuit-priest". June 18, 1949 I, with twenty other Jesuits, stretched face down in the sanctuary while the litanies were chanted. It felt so right to be in that position begging God to forgive me and to do what had to be done to consecrate me His priest. Then Carinal Cushing imposed hands on me and I was a priest.

The three hour ceremony on Saturday and the first Mass Sunday were deeply moving experiences and transformed my life. Definitely etched in my consciousness was the realization that I was a priest. Every priestly act and every response in faith to me as priest deepened the etching. A new period of fervor welled up. Celebrating Mass, especially for the people, preaching, hearing confessions, spiritual direction inspired me with the challenge to be what I seemed. Material activities expressive of my priesthood came to occupy much of my day.

The third stage of becoming spanned about thirteen years. A fourth year of theology at Weston, tertianship or third year of noviceship in Belgium, two years of philosophy in Rome, and about ten years of teaching philosophy during which I also helped at the local parish on weekends. The first four of these years were simply an extension of the previous period of formation, clearly preparation to be and to do. Yet something distinctive was present: I was a priest. I kept growing in familiarity with this fact. Wherever I went, even when traveling and staying in hotels, an essential detail concerned where and when I would say Mass. I believe that the practice of a devout Mass did much to pre serve my vocation. Even when prayer was regularly neglected and fervor was low, I had the daily occasion of encountering God and facing the state of my heart. Celebrating Mass in the parishes and preaching likewise provided keen reminders. Often it was a consolation to rea lize I was not preaching myself but Jesus Christ. Other wise I would not have had the courage to preach. Still the demand to put my life in accord with what I was preaching proved purgative.

Travel liberated me, of course, as it does most. My puritanical stuffiness was partially, at least, sloughed off. In the same process self respect grew as well as patriotism. Roots were perceived in the family of man as I tasted the achievements of man in art, architecture and historical monuments. Entwined in these European roots were the roots of my Christian heritage as well. Rome and the living Pope vitalized my Catholic union and pride. The warm reception received in Jesuit communities in six different countries as well as intimate living with fellow Jesuits from all over the world, including China, India, South America and the Iron Curtain countries, increased my love for, and pride in, the Society of Jesus.

The tertianship was designed as a "school of affection" to offset the effect of long years of preparation and dry, intellectualizing study. It was, as the name suggests (tertius annus) a third year of noviceship, a time for prayer. The high point once again was the thirty-day retreat. I went through, in a more mature way, the same series of experiences leading to joyful recommitment to Christ. I prayed much during the year, caught deeper insight into the spirit of the Society through study of the Constitutions, discovered the articulation of the Spiritual Exercises, but experienced no lasting conversion or transformation. Possibly the fact I was assigned, that I did not freely elect, to make tertianship led me to enter it as "the next thing" to be done and so lessened the impact of the year's experiences. No doubt, however, it did deepen my vocation.

For the most part the courses at Rome and my own work were depth probings within my own tradition. Hence no great awakening. Some valuable things were going on at the university but I did not have the energy to get into them. Much as I appreciated being in Rome and sharing with inspiring Jesuits from all over the world, the constant attrition of a strange land and strange customs had a wearing and wearying effect. Before the first year was over I had burned myself out and took off for Ireland where the doctor put me to pasture for the entire summer, diagnosing nervous exhaustion. My last year I confined my efforts to essentials, determined to finish my thesis. This I did and returned home August 1953 in time to make my retreat prior to final vows on the 15th.

The Society had invested seventeen years to prepare
me to teach philosophy to younger Jesuits at Weston College, our seminary. And I felt anything but ready. I
was to present the reasoned proofs of the existence of
God, explain how we can speak about God and what we can
know by reason about His nature and His relation to us.
The objective was to comprehend the problems and penetrate the solutions, not to present the history of
thought on these topics or expose some philsopher's position. After twenty years of struggling with these
problems I still feel inadequate. Obviously I found
the demands sobering. These questions were not merely
academic. They concerned the prelude to faith and religion.

I came to grips with radical contemporary denial of
my basic positions in a course I gave on Logical Posi-
tivism and Linguistic Analysis. I widened my background
by courses, two semesters at Harvard and another semester
at New York University where I sat in on two courses by
A. G. N. Flew, an English analyst and atheist. Attendance at the Institute for Religion in an Age of Science
exposed me to full-blown naturalism.

While I worked to establish my professional compe-
tence as a philosopher I began to exercise my priesthood more directly by preaching and directing retreats.
I also became a regular assistant at St. Julia's, the
local parish. This meant hearing confessions Saturday afternoon and evening, two Masses on Sunday and
help whenever an emergency occurred. Not only did I
enjoy exercising my priesthood for the people, not only
did I develop some close, meaningful friendships, but
also this involvement laid bare the relationship between refined speculation and ordinary living. The
challenge of naturalism I met in my studies found echoes
in the lives of the people.

At the same time significant social relations were
being established. My sister had had her first baby a
month after I had left for Belgium. So on my return
Marybeth was almost three. I joined my sister's family,
as it were, sharing with her and her husband the growth
and development of their family of four. Many dimensions of human living found expression in this relationship. It kept my feet on the ground, providing a practical view of the problems of ordinary living. Contact
with my brother and his family and with other relatives
contributed in the same way as did friendships developed with other families.

Perhaps that indiscernible point at which it was possible to say 'I am Jesuit-priest', instead of 'I am becoming Jesuit-priest' was reached through a climactic experience with one of these families. Acquaintance began, as I recall, at the baptism of their third child. Acquaintance rapidly became friendship and a warm love developed as they allowed me to share so much in their lives. I shared in their pleasures, I shared in their anxieties and sufferings. Years wove many binding threads. Then the wife left the Church, taking the children with her. The years of warmly shared friendship made this a deeply upsetting experience, shaking my own faith. One often heard, even at that time, of people giving up their faith and while it struck one as sad, it did not upset. But that someone I care for so much and whose intelligence and integrity I respected should deliberately walk away from the Church was entirely different. I found myself asking, am I wrong? Have I been mistaken? Is there really a God? Is Jesus Christ divine? These two basic questions preoccupied me. Over and over again I faced their challenge. The traditional proofs for the existence of God which I had been teaching now came to life. Are they truly valid? Do they satisfy me? I found them far from adequate in my genuine struggle. They did, however, provide a framework. Perhaps it was the faith and love of friends who did not even know my anguish which fleshed them out, allowing me to catch the needed insights and to respond in love.

Peace returned with the prayerful reaffirmation of my faith. And I vividly realized the need of keeping my faith green and fresh. It may be that this experience made me shape up. Certainly I situate that first level when I actually had succeeded in structuring a meaningful life about a year or so after this experience.

About the time peace was settling in other friendships took seed or started to blossom. All the time, of course, quiet friendships within the Society had been nurtured. I felt I belonged to the community.

I am sobered as I say that it was in my middle forties before my life could be described as being, rather than becoming, meaningful. Still maybe that should not surprise since I was thirty-six when I finished my formal education and began my professional role as teacher. The entire process had, of course, very definitely been meaningful, but in terms of becoming, not of being. To reach a sense of confidence in a field like philosophy and ease in the role as priest ten years or more does not seem excessively slow. I imagine it takes that long to become at ease in marriage or/and as a doctor.

I was fortunate in the timing, coming of age as it were before the Church and civil upheavals of the late sixties. These brought painful experiences and profound changes. But I knew who I was and was able to change from one level of being meaningful to another. I have sympathy for the young as they struggle to find themselves in this period of change. Painful as the conflicts have been I am beginning to be grateful as I recognize that they have made me more alive and helped me to grow as never before.

What prompts me to claim that about this time the process of structuring meaning into my life was over? At some point it was no longer accurate to say I was becoming Jesuit-priest, for indeed I had become, I was a Jesuit-priest. I do not mean to suggest that something striking happened: even now I can designate the date in only roughest fashion. I was not conscious of suddenly being different. Neither do I want to suggest that change or growth ceased. By no means.

I am attempting to do what the young cannot do: indicate the difference between the meaning in life based on hope, on becoming and the meaning in a life in which one has truly become one and whole. Some may dispute the point, convinced that all of life is a becoming. For them the chase, the struggle is the goal. I do not wish to argue the point. I merely describe my experience: I now am one and whole, I am consciously one, my desires harmonized under the dominant desire to love and serve God as Jesuit priest. I find life meaningful and happy. When I entered the Society I <u>hoped</u> to be a Jesuit-priest, I hoped this would prove meaningful. To be in the process of becoming a Jesuit-priest was indeed meaningful--meaningful in hope, in preparation. But to be in the process of becoming is not to be. And I testify that the consciousness of being one and whole as Jesuit priest differs significantly from that of becoming Jesuit-priest.

If I start from present consciousness and summon to memory the changes I have experienced since the mid-sixties I recognize how significantly I have changed in my attitudes, my perspective, my life-style. But I see myself as remaining substantially what I had become, a Jesuit-priest. Through these changes I lived my Jesuit priesthood in different ways. I say this in keen awareness of the pain, the conflict, the soul searching involved in the process of these changes. Nor do I feel the changes are over. I sense I may be on the verge of further and most significant transformations. Not only is the very character of my community being changed this year, but the whole Society of Jesus has just finished a world-wide self-examination and updating, issuing in a document inviting me to challenge radically my objectives and lifestyle. Again I see these anticipated changes making me more fully what I already am. So the changes since the mid-sixties and those anticipated are from being Jesuit-priest on one level to being Jesuit-priest on another level. But if I let my memory run back before the sixties the difference I detect between what I am now and what I was then is far greater than the differences effected by these more recent changes. This is truer the further back I go. I find it impossible to describe this difference. But is is as real as the difference between a recognized concert pianist and the same person a year before he was ready for his first concert. This imaginary person may be pictured as desiring to be a concert pianist much as I desired to be a Jesuit priest. Commitment to becoming such projected us in our respective directions. We practiced, we prepared--there was no guarantee either of us would succeed in being what we desired. Time, experiences, development shaped us to approximations of our projected roles. For some time it is clear that he is not a concert pianist, he is a promising prospect. At another point it is beyond question that he has arrived: he is a concert pianist. It is impossible to discern exactly when he ceased to be promising and actually arrived at being a concert pianist. My entire Jesuit life has been meaningful, but for years I found meaning in preparing to be a Jesuit priest, just as this pianist found his years of preparing meaningful. At some point I "had it all together" and meaning was securely structured into my life. I moved with ease as Jesuit priest.

I am finding this explanation difficult ultimately because becoming can only be understood in relation to being. The process of my becoming a Jesuit-priest makes sense only in terms of what being a Jesuit priest has meant. Being Jesuit-priest, of course, not only permits the profound changes referred to above but also substantial restructuring. Friends have decided to leave the Society and the priesthood and seem to have succeeded in structuring meaningful lives as husband-fathers.

At some indiscernible point, then, I had become
one and whole. I had grown comfortable in my different
roles as my various desires blended with my dominant desire to love God as Jesuit-priest. Most of my time and
energy were devoted to specifically Jesuit and priestly
activities. Most importantly I had become this certain
kind of person. As the doctor finds fulfillment not in
doing doctor-things, but in being a doctor, so I had so
harmonized my life that I was at ease in most circumstances. At a party I was priest. On the altar I was
human. At a philosophy convention I was priestly philosopher. In the pulpit I was philosopher-priest. I had
indeed not become distinguished as Jesuit or priest or
philosopher. Yet even in mediocrity I had come to be
consciously one and whole, at ease being me as Jesuit
priest.

Unlike a subordinating desire the dominant desire
allows indulgence in other desires unless they conflict
with it. I pursued my other desires as I felt their ap-
peal--friendship, literature, theater, sports, tele-
vision, recreation in general. Various dimensions of
my person found expression in these desires and suitable refreshment of spirit was provided. Often, I fear,
I ignored or in self-deception denied actual conflict
between certain desires and my dominant desire. As a
result commitment was watered down and I failed to become as one and whole as possible. When, however, the
delusions revealed themselves for what they were, for
the most part I made hard choices under the guidance
of my dominant desire as a negative norm.

At this point in my reflections I began to experience an excitement similar to that which the analysis
of my overarching meaning had stirred up. I had re-
lived, letting my life unfold before me, the strange,
dialectical stages through which I became consciously
one, through which I became the distinctive person I
am. The desire to be Jesuit-priest had to come to
birth, be nurtured, bring to death the simple pious boy
so a new man could be born. In this new man the desire
had to face the risks of being overthrown by newly
awakened human desires in my maturity. It had to sink
roots and permeate more and more of my life--patiently,
slowly and never with guarantee of success. Gradually
it grew so securely enmeshed, so dominantly appealing
that it harmonized all other desires.

I had found that being Jesuit priest fulfilled all
three criteria I had discovered as indicative of a dominant desire. Surely it functioned as a negative norm

among my other desires and commanded more and more of my time and energy. More significantly it pointed to and explained the distinctive person I had become. Desire welled up from a sense of realized wholeness and from perceiving the sharp features of the self I had become. Desire to live as that self. Desire rooted in the personal history laid out before my eyes and enlivened by amazement and gratitude at the providential control of the effects of what happened in my life. I felt called to be that self.

I know I had been very fortunate in life. Everything had come together. I could not have reached this wholeness in the harmonization of desires unless my overarching meaning had effectively undergird the entire enterprise. And at this point mine was significantly operative, shaping me as a Christian humanist. Basic needs were provided for by the Society. My vow of poverty had liberated me from material concerns, all I owned or earned went to the Society. Although my various activities, teaching, preaching, directing retreats, do bring in definite sums of money, I never see it. The evaluation of what I do is not in terms of dollars but in terms of the Jesuit apostolic efforts.

I loved everything I did. Indeed I have been "doing my own thing" for a long time. I am constantly traveling in mind, not among places, but among ideas, intellectual problems. I enjoy the challenge of young minds, hoping to open them to the truths that shape their lives, but discovering in turn the roots of my own positions as I try to show how these positions grow out of their experienced truth and values. I love to hear confessions, offer Mass with and for people, preach; I love the spiritual challenge to honesty and growth I experience in directing retreats.

In all of these activities I enjoyed considerable freedom, leisure to prepare and responsibility. Friendships warmed my heart, refreshed me, kept me human and alive. Habits structured my life, though unfortunately, I was not sufficiently sensitive to their shackling effects on my spirit and the spirits of other especially the seminarians. Good fortune and the caring and good sense of friends, however, had built a rhythm of activities into my life that kept it vital. Life felt very meaningful and I was tempted to forego further analysis. Living is more important than understanding. And after all I already knew by intuition as well as lived experience that I was right. Still I had spread out my life in such detail in order to be able to veri-

fy my analysis of the constitutive elements of a meaningful life. If the analysis permitted me to articulate the link between the pain and the loss of meaning
I experienced I would consider the analysis confirmed.
I was now in a position to face this test.

CHAPTER SEVEN

PAIN and the Loss of Meaning

Life at this point did indeed feel very meaningful and the idea of further analysis had the taste of futility. I experienced no need of analysis: intuitively I knew how pain linked with my loss of meaning. Besides, serious doubts oozed up whether any of my analysis would be able to help others at all. Is not the vocation, the life of a Jesuit priest so removed from ordinary experience that few could identify with my reactions? Would insights into the structure of meaning in my life as a Jesuit priest be judged simply invalid for secular lives? Would my very language make the account suspect? Do my efforts to reveal my religious attitudes have the ring of pious rhetoric? Do readers sense I am preaching instead of thinking aloud? Do I sound inauthentic, unreal? Such doubts forced me to probe my heart and intentions. I found I could honestly say that not a single word have I written in a 'sweet', 'pious' mood or from an intention to preach. My struggle has been to be accurate, to find words which rang true to my experiences and captured my insights. I know how an unfamiliar rhetoric or idiom can sound artificial, insincere. I have tried to be utterly sincere and as genuine as insight and pen permit. While I remain convinced that my life is based upon the truth (and I am certain that man's happiness depends upon discovering and living the truth) I can honestly say that I have revealed my beliefs only for their bearing upon the structure of the meaning in my life. I have not been preaching or arguing them.

In my heart I could answer to the suspicion of being inauthentic or 'preachy'. I simply had to trust that my sincerity would be recognized. But the other doubt persisted: has my experience as a Jesuit priest anything to say to those living married, secular lives? My assumption that insight into my experience definitely would be valid for any life was now shaken. I felt forced to take another hard look at my analysis. Insight had uncovered the structure of meaning in my life. Were the final structure and the process of structuring sufficiently distinct from the religious content to be valid for other contexts and other contents? A little reflection let me see that it was not the structure but the process of structuring which prompted this doubt.

Recognition of the need of the overarching meaning and the harmonization of desires, the two essential constitutive elements of a meaningful life, sprang from seeing the person as a moment of experiencing, a drive-to-be moved on by multiple desires. No restriction there. The spectrum of world-views competing for the role of overarching meaning makes clear we are not talking religion. As for the harmonization of desires I had illustrated both the subordinating and the dominant desire with secular examples. The other elements of the structure of a meaningful life such as expression of a sufficient number of the dimensions of the drive-to-be, wise selection of activities, not to mention the relation of the means of providing for basic needs, obviously are distinct from religious content. No, the doubt did not arise from the structure I had uncovered.

To capture the process by which meaning became structured into my life had proved far more subtle, far more difficult than to intuit from within the actual structure that made it meaningful. What had prompted this subtle, concentrated effort had been the hope of helping young people to develop meaningful lives. If I could uncover the salient steps by which my life had been successfully made meaningful, perhaps, I felt, the young could glean hints for their own projects. Hope had initiated such reflections, but these reflections were finally generating doubt. For as reflective analysis laid bare the religious values and inspirations intertwined in my development, it risked turning off the young. Not only might the language seem inauthentic, pious rhetoric to young ears, but many youth, unable to identify with such values, might fail to discern the natural human aspects of my experiences they very definitely do share. I suddenly had to ask myself: am I in fact sufficiently attentive to these human aspects?

I pulled the film of recollections from the shelf and re-ran it, searching for those shared, distinctively human aspects in the process by which meaning became structured into my life. The noviceship experiences immediately provided a serious challenge. Few, it seemed, could identify with these. The intense experience of the thirty-day retreat is not paralleled in many lives. It is not easy to imagine what transpires when one has blocked up the normal desires for marriage, wealth and control of one's plans. Interiorized sensitivity to the presence of God and to underlying motivations in conduct and attitudes is not commonly experienced. Fellow religious would, of course, recognize how ordinary all this is. Non-believers on the other hand could at

most respect my sincerity and try to cut through the
religious claims to the psychological changes claimed,
hard put not to put me down as deluded. But even devout believers, unless they lived an interior, spiritual life, might be bewildered trying to follow what
happened to me.

Yet every human experience can be identified with
through analogy with one's own. Varying degrees of ab-
straction reveal the similarity of experiences. Thus
a focus upon my psychological reactions, abstracting
from the religious content, should allow anyone to perceive how much we have in common. This first stage in
my process of becoming a Jesuit priest involved a powerful, emotional upheaval as I changed the orientation
of my life. Instead of continuing along the direction
in which I had been trained, I deliberately chose a new
way of life. The depth of upheaval required to effect
the reorientation will be in proportion to the degree
of change. The upheaval in my life was very like a conversion. But I would also liken it to the emotional upheaval of early marriage as two individuals face the
challenge to change from living for oneself to living
for one another. Taken abstractly my noviceship experience involved serious, deliberate choice to reorient
my life, emotional upheaval, followed by deepened intellectual conviction and definite practices to establish habitual responses appropriate to the new orientation. So described the first stage of the structuring
of meaning into my life should not seem strange. Most
meaningful lives will involve a similar process.

I began to feel easier about the doubt raised
about the process I went through to structure meaning
into my life. So long as the noviceship experience,
the first stage of the process, could be recognized
as similar to serious change in anyone's life, the second and third stages should raise little difficulty.
It is hardly foreign to human experience to live intensely under a subordinating desire during early fervor of a new commitment but then through familiarity,
routine and the ordinary demands of life to slip into
mediocrity. If few could identify with my long retreat experiences, my desire to give myself to Christ's
kingdom, most could understand the effect of my introduction to lobster, scotch and cigarettes. Most could
resonate with my remorse as I faced the challenge before ordination: what have you done with the years?

During the second stage I did indeed grow, humanly
and even spiritually. But the compelling power of the

desire to be Jesuit priest dissipated before the appeal
of my other desires. It continued to harmonize my life,
but as a dominant, not a subordinating desire. In fact
it was almost overthrown by the desire for marriage.
It faced many risks even in the protective structure of
a religious lifestyle. I reaffirmed my choice with
clearer vision of the sacrifice involved in at least
two critical decisions. Many a person at thirty-three
must have experienced similar challenges to his marriage or to his professional commitment. He probably
feels fortunate or blessed if he succeeded as well as
I in reaffirming his original commitment. Loyalty and
perseverance are necessary for any worthwhile achievement. And since most of us suffer in our ideals under
the attrition of life, it is not hard to understand that
life can be meaningful even in mediocrity.

The third stage of my development of a meaningful
life is probably the easiest to identify with. Within
a framework of the ordinary I became more at ease as
Jesuit-priest-professor. Friendships expanded, I man-
aged to establish a blend and rhythm of activities expressive of what I was. Certainly anyone who has
achieved meaning in life easily understands what happened to me.

The doubts dissolved but I still had to force myself to work out in detail what I intuitively realize,
-how pain was linked with my loss of meaning. For a few
years I had been living a life meaningful in being, not
just in becoming, a Jesuit priest. I had not become
distinguished as religious or priest or philosopher or
teacher. Still even in the mediocrity due to my failure to live as completely as possible the Jesuit priest
I was, my life was genuinely meaningful. Pain struck
and my life became non-meaningful. Why?

As I described in the opening chapter intense pain
forced a profound, emotional challenge to the existence
of a God who would permit such pain. Christ's crucifixion and friends' love provided counter-emotional evidence, thus preventing denial of God. But the pain and
the challenge made me cease to count on Him. God was
not swept out of my life but He no longer was important.
The central, pivotal factor of my overarching meaning,
Christian humanism, as well as of my dominant desire,
Jesuit priest, became muted. No wonder life became
non-meaningful.

As a drive-to-be moving under the appeal of desires
my life had been structured under the overarching mean-

94

ing of Christian humanism. God, the keystone of this overarching meaning, had in turn so permeated my life that love of God came to function as my dominant desire harmonizing the activites which made up my life as a Jesuit priest.

As a result of the pain I no longer desired God. I did not deny God, for then I would have been defining myself as rejecting belief in God. I would have become angry with my past deception and been driven to restructure my life or I would have despaired as life became, not non-meaningful, but meaningless. No, it was not denial. I did not hate God. I did not desire anything more than God. Desire for God just ceased.

Since God's existence was not denied the overarching meaning did not come down. I do not recall any sense of absurdity. I just seem to have withdrawn my attention from any question of meaning beyond the present. As God became unimportant so did anything beyond immediate desires. Thus the experience in pain affected my overarching meaning by forcing me to withdraw attention to it and to focus on immediate desires. But immediate desires ceased to appeal as the shock affected my dominant desire.

My desires had been harmonized under my dominant desire of love of God concretized in desire to serve Him as Jesuit priest. I no longer counted on God: how then could I truly desire to be Jesuit priest? To restate an earlier synthetic summary: I can act only if I am. I can be only if I am one. I can act with meaning and desire only if I am meaningful to myself. I can be meaningful to myself only if I am consciously one. I can be consciously one only if I am harmonized as one under a subordinating or dominant desire. Once the emotional shock of pain made God unimportant to me my dominant desire ceased to harmonize my conscious life. I ceased to be consciously one, ceased to be meaningful to myself. Hence I simply could not act with meaning or desire.

This result becomes more clearly articulated if you reflect upon the material activities which make up the life of a Jesuit priest. No one can just love God! Oliver and Vincent, the two characters I used to illustrate the way a dominant desire functions, and I are drives-to-be in flesh. Love of God can be only one element in our being, even though it can permate all other elements. Suppose that love of God were to be truly the dominant desire for Oliver and Vincent, God calling them to express this love in becoming husband-father. Such a commitment would involve particular activities. The formal element would be love of God which would find expression in the material element, the set of human, secular activities of living together, working, raising a family and all that these imply. My dominant desire to love God leading to becoming Jesuit priest became incarnated in a set of material activities far different, most in principle directly related to God

If you look back to my "Autobiography of a Dominant Desire" you will observe that my life came to be made up of two kinds of material activities: those ordered to nurturing union with God such as prayer, spiritual reading, and reception of the Sacraments; and those undertaken as service of God through His Church for men such as preaching, teaching, celebrating Mass, hearing confessions, directing retreats. Unlike the material activities proper to the married lives of Oliver and Vincent all the material activities proper to my life as Jesuit priest draw their meaning directly from their relation to God. If I could not count on God, the soul, the raison d'etre of all the material activities of my life died.

I did, however, continue to exist and so I had to act. To act I had to follow some desire. Thus the me as simply a living being was distinct from me as a person structured in a unique, distinctive way as a Jesuit priest. Although I, as person, could not act with meaning, habits carried me from need to need. I rose, I dressed, I ate, I read a bit, watched TV. But I did not want to do anything. Spontaneity vanished. I ceased to be meaningful to myself and in that sense I ceased to be. In a limbo state nothing called to me. Life was non-meaningful.

At this point I felt I had sufficiently articulated the link between my experience of pain and the loss of meaning in my life. The very fact I needed to refer only to the effect of pain on my overarching meaning and my dominant desire reveals that these two (of the seven) elements are essentially constitutive of the meaningful life. And the ease with which the structure of meaning in life I had developed proved able to explain my loss of meaning was further evidence of its truth. But I felt tempted to imagine the effect of a similar experience in pain on Oliver or Vincent whose lives were structured under a different dominant desire. Would he have reacted as I did?

Recall that God was very real to Oliver and Vincent, definitely functioning as the keystone in their overarching meaning. Furthermore desire, love of God was significant among their desires, even though desire to be husband-father it was which functioned to harmonize their lives as dominant desire. If pain then were to render God unimportant to one of them, there can be no question that meaning in his life would be seriously affected. Immediately his overarching meaning would be affected. Probably as with me it would fade into the background. The question of the ultimate meaning of life would not be asked. Instead he too would focus upon immediate desires.

Of course if the whole no longer seems meaningful (which is what the overarching meaning effects) it seems impossible that immediate desires would seem meaningful-- if one allowed the question to be asked. So I imagine that pain would temporarily at least erase the question. Thus like me he would focus upon immediate desires.

Now I presume that the loss of, disappointment in, any significant desire would seriously affect one's life. Since God functioned prominently in the constellation of his desires I presume Oliver or Vincent would find meaning definitely affected. But being husband-father, his dominant desire, would still appeal, still function to keep his oneness and identity. Sad though he would be he would be consciously one and his material activities would continue to appeal.

We can push this analysis further by imagining an Oliver or Vincent for whom love of God is truly his dominant desire leading him to express this love as husband and father. If pain so invaded his body that he no longer counted on God, then indeed would meaning in his life be lost. But the reason would lie in the dissolution of his oneness and self-identity, not in the loss of appeal in the material activities. Without being consciously one none of his normal desires would function. But I would assume that the material activities would retain at least some of their intrinsic appeal. He would by no means be happy. But the need of providing for basic needs would, I imagine, move him into action. Sexual expression, conjugal and parental love, though not so keenly felt would probably evoke response.

The difference I am trying to bring out between meaning in my life and that in such an Oliver or Vincent with regard to material activities can be underscored by

97

imagining the original Oliver or Vincent if either were
to lose his wife through death or separation. This would
directly affect his dominant desire of being husband-father. Not only would meaning go out of his life because
he ceased to be consciously one, but the material activities of his life would be directly affected. Some simply
would cease, others such as work would probably lose all
appeal since their formal element would have been lost.

Surely that suffices. What I had known intuitively I had succeeded in articulating in detail: the link
between pain and the loss of meaning in my life. It was
almost like empirical verification to find that, under
challenge, my intuitive certainty that my insights explained the loss of meaning could meet the test of step
by step articulation.

How I wish I had discovered more than the structure of meaning in life. Last night a young man let me
know how lost he is. I am able to resonate with his
sadness, his emptiness, the lack of orientation in his
life. I am even able to pick out some of the reasons
at the root of his mood, a mood that has lasted a long
while. His overarching meaning has ceased to be operative so that conviction has been sapped that life as a
whole has meaning. Although he wants to marry somehow
I sense he does not realize that is the dominant desire
around which he can build his life. He has been going
two years with the girl he desires to marry but anything definite about marriage has been avoided. For
not only has he another year to go in a professional
program but he is by no means sure he wants that profession. Yes my insights allow me to pinpoint certain
needs, but how limited I felt when he almost cried, asking "where do I start?"

I am a philosopher, not a counselor. I have sought
to understand the true, constitutive elements of a meaningful life which must underlie any technique or procedure to create or to restore meaning. But I am not
equipped to work out any such technique. Still possibly I could at least put him on the road and in the
right direction.

In chapter three I revealed a process by which I
discovered what it was about me that I needed an overarching meaning. I think I will have him repeat this
process. Let him go into himself and realize that all
he is, all he possesses is this moment of experiencing.
Soon he will recognize that the moment is structured by
past experiences and future desires. As he reflects
upon his personal history and the actual desires which

move him on, he should grow in the appreciation that he is unique and free. Somehow I sense he is not free enough, he has not truly chosen to create his self. Meaning will be so dependent upon his exercise of responsible freedom. But hopefully also he will recognize the need to ask whether the series of desires, the whole, makes sense. Having been raised a Catholic he probably will recognize Christian humanism as the overarching meaning he has lived under. Now he will have to decide for himself--under grace--whether he can embrace such beliefs. Bracketing the moral question of culpability in loss of faith I would say that only if he personally commits himself to such a life or positively replaces it can he reestablish meaning. I can make suggestions how to proceed, but the mystery of God's action and free will enters at this point: only he can decide.

If he rises to freedom and to a decision on the overarching meaning, he may feel so excited and unified that he may delude himself that everything is cleared up. Actually he still must face the challenge of harmonizing his diverse desires. Since he does not seem any more than I the heroic type, capable of committing himself to one subordinating desire, his task is to select the dominant desire which will make him the kind of person he is to become. If he can accept that the self he is to be is his to create, choosing to marry this girl--even if the marriage must be postponed--will harmonize his desires, give meaning to all he does with a strength and delight such as he has never experienced.

Is she really the right woman for him? Will she truly want to be wife and mother as he develops being husband-father? There is no guarantee. Only sensitive, wise assessment can make the risk reasonable. But risk, commitment there must be. A responsible decision will be needed to bring harmony into his life.

But another serious decision faces him. Does he really want this profession he is training for? The unhappiness he is experiencing, the lack of drive and achievement compared to his college years create doubt. Personally I believe he should finish the training, and vigorously,--understanding he remains free to engage in the field or not. It is not psychologically healthy to fail to complete such a serious undertaking. He must, however, remain free to follow the profession or not. If his life is to be fully meaningful and happy, the career must blend easily with his domi-

nant desire. In principle a person deliberating about
work is seeking three things: activity which allows
for his talents and inclinations, work which is worthwhile, and work which will provide for basic needs and
other desires. So often in our culture one or other of
these aspects must be sacrificed. In our technocratic
society the actual priorities for most are: work which
makes enough money to provide for needs and desire, then
activity which appeals and engages one's talents, and
only third that which is worthwhile.

So my young friend should once again rise to responsible freedom and really choose his career. I do
not believe he made a genuine choice when he applied
for this professional program. I intend to recommend
the testing services at the university to help him become sharply aware of his aptitudes, inclinations and
possible careers. Friends who know him well and people
actually following the different careers can provide
light. But there are no guarantees in this area either.
If he has entered seriously into the process of tasting
what he is and what actually moves him he will be prepared to use such aids. Four general suggestions: let
him become sensitive to what he genuinely enjoys, to
his genuine values and convictions; let him remain true
to his own judgments and feelings; let him know that
the choice is his alone; let him choose as he judges
God is leading him to choose.

It seems to me that my young friend might well recapture meaning for his life by going in such directions.
It will, of course, only be the meaning of becoming,
the meaning of hope. As it took years before I could
say "I am Jesuit priest professor and it is good", so
time, much time will be required before the process
of becoming gives birth to the wholeness of the person
he is to be. Love, for instance, does not grow without
sharing, without sacrifice and discipline. Success
and ease in one's career requires much of the same.
Wisdom, sensitivity must be exercised. Unless a sufficient number of the dimensions of his self are given
expression, dullness can enter. Hopefully he, with his
wife, will establish habits providing for all these aspects of their lives. If they are wise they will, however, remain sensitive to the possible shackling rather
than liberating effects of such habits. Happiness does
not just happen, even though so many factors are contingent, providential. One has to keep alive, freely, responsibly creating the self in all circumstances.

These efforts to apply my insights to my young

friend's needs encouraged me to believe that my work may indeed prove useful to others. At the very least they have served as a way of summarizing the key element of meaning which I had discovered. If the analysis of meaning is, as I believe, true, then perhaps persons gifted with a more practical outlook may be led to develop techniques suitable for guiding people to create or to restore meaning in lives.